VAIDYA CINTAMANI
AN ANCIENT MEDICAL TEXT OF SOUTHERN INDIA

SRINIVASARAO PEDAPROLU

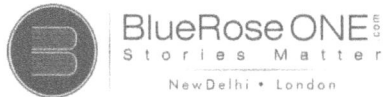

BLUEROSE PUBLISHERS
India | U.K.

Copyright © Srinivasarao Pedaprolu 2025

All rights reserved by author. No part of this publication may be reproduced, stored in a retrieval system or transmitted in any form or by any means, electronic, mechanical, photocopying, recording or otherwise, without the prior permission of the author. Although every precaution has been taken to verify the accuracy of the information contained herein, the publisher assume no responsibility for any errors or omissions. No liability is assumed for damages that may result from the use of information contained within.

BlueRose Publishers takes no responsibility for any damages, losses, or liabilities that may arise from the use or misuse of the information, products, or services provided in this publication.

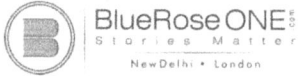

For permissions requests or inquiries regarding this publication, please contact:

BLUEROSE PUBLISHERS
www.BlueRoseONE.com
info@bluerosepublishers.com
+91 8882 898 898
+4407342408967

ISBN: 978-93-6783-073-4

Cover design: Daksh
Typesetting: Tanya Raj Upadhyay

First Edition: January 2025

PREFACE

Medical science is always progressive with the advent of various experiences of the physicians and such progress in medical science is endless. New research developments in the field of medicine have been recorded and also published by many a number of scholars. The local contributions in this way have either supported the dictum of Ayurveda or added to the armamentarium of the techniques of the disease management. It is incumbent on the successive generations to observe in retrospect to what factor and factors contributed. Unfortunately such efforts are not given due credit and adopted by the so called elite practitioners who just believe in brihatrayee and blind towards other valuable literatures. Vaidyachintamani can be placed in the foremost prominence just because the versatility pluralism and holistic approach adopted in the compilation of the text. Many andhrite practitioners of south India are benefitted by following this work. In this book "Vaidyacintamani an ancient medical text of southern India" I tried to elicit how the author was differing with brihatrayee (Caraka, Susruta and Vagbhata) with respect to diseases clinical conditions, treatments and also what were the priorities given etc. Other factors like religious conditions prevailed in those days, the status of the physician in the society, his role in the promotion of the ethics in the society, mode of drug administration, commonly used drugs, dose schedule, what measurements were used, social customs etc., are described.

ABOUT THE BOOK

Author of Vaidya cintamani Indrakanthi vallabhacharya belongs to medieval Andhra desa (southern India), a great Ayurveda vaidya of his times. This statement supported by below mentioned sloka.

श्रिवत्सगोत्रतिलक : जगद्वैद्यपितामह : अमरेश्वर भत्तस्य प्रियसोङ्गुनोन्नत:
तद्सावल्लभेन्द्रेण क्रियते हितकारक :वैद्यचिन्तामनिर्नाम भैषज्य ग्रन्थ उत्तम :

He introduced himself in the introductory verse and the colophon of his medical work Vaidya Chintamani that he was well versed in all sastras, jagatvaidya pitamaha, an eminent scholar in the science of medicine and versed in all scholarship and knowledge.

He was the son of Amareswara bhattaraka. Though he introduced himself as a great poet, we do not find any other literary works on his name. We do not find any information regarding his native place or date. It is thought That Vallabhacharya might have trained in the kingdom of Vidyanagara (Vijayanagara) and belongs to Andhradesa basing on the mentioning of places, articles and the words he used most often in the text.

The book Vaidya cintamani considered as bhashajya grantha uttama and is widely referred book by Andhra practitioners since consisting efficacious formulations which are proven to be clinically highly effective.

Vallabhacharya's work was quoted by many scholars on medicine, Basavaraju, who lived between AD 1450-1525 and also author of Vaidya yoga ratnavali a famous book of

Ayurveda referred to Vaidya Chintamni. Hence it is clear that Vaidya chintamani is quite earlier than Basavarajeeyamu and Vaidya yoga Ratnavali. Vaidyachintamani a compendium of efficacious formulations, therapeutic procedures, dietetic advises hence became a source for the later works on medicine .

Vaidya chintamni, a very authentic work on Ayurveda written by Indra Kanthi Vallabha charya who composed this work in Sanskrit but script was in telugu, hence was not popular among the other parts of the country just because it was not published in devanagari script of Sanskrit.

There are different manuscripts of vaidya chintamani available in different places viz:GOML13095 manuscript available in Government oriental manuscript library, Madras in kannada language. In the same library GOML13361 to 13374 and 13096 to 13097 manuscripts are available in telugu language. In govt oriental library, Mysore the following manuscripts are available VIZOLM2054, OLM168 and OLM283.script of these manuscripts is in telugu and kannada. Apart from these manuscripts of vaidya chintamani and some more manuscripts are available in Sarswatimahal library, Tanjore, tamilnadu, Bhadarkar oriental research institute pune, maharashtra, and also in Govt oriental manuscrpipts library and research institute, Hyderabad. Later in. the end of 19th AD it is published in telugu language in Hinduratnakara, Mudrakshara shala, Madras by pidugu Subbaramayya and sons and after that by vavilla Ramasastrulu and sons, Madras in 1952. The importance of Vaidyacintamani can be elucidated by its inclusion under drugs and cosmetics act 1940.

Total contents of this book is divided into 25 number of vilasa. Further each vilasa described in the form of different prakarana.Though the slokas are described in the sanskrit but the script of the sloka is in telugu. This book is started with mangalacharana by praying all the important deities of Hindu . He has written this book by picking up best recipes from various sources of Ayurveda and also added of his own from his experience. He was selfless and kept no secret in disclosing the very efficacious formulations to the up coming physicians.

In this book we find elaborative description about Nadi pariksha (pulse examination), though this appears similar to Nadipariksha mentioned by Sarangadhara etc., but its description in vaidyacintamani altogether differs. In the preparation of formulations of medicine there is extensive use of animal products like matsya pitta (bile of fish), mahisha ghrta (buffalo ghee) etc., which were used for bhavana, mardana etc.

In this book apart from karmavipaka, jyotissastraabhipraya, causative factors (nidana), symptoms (lakshanas), mode of occurrence (samprapti) of diseases and also its curability, incurability.pathya, apthya and treatment is explained. The treatment of karma vipaka generally consisted of daiva vyapasraya chikitsa (worshipping god etc) along with usual principles of treatment advised for each disease.

Generally the treatment i.e the drugs are administered in the form of kashaya, rasayoga, curna, vati, avalehya, ghrita, taila, nasya, anjana vidhi, dhuma and lepa for each disease .He also advises to undergo relevant panchakarma procedures.

In this book, we get description of procedures of dravya sodhana, bhasma preparation and about different types of yantras and maana (weights and measurements).

The book thus designed to fulfill every knowledge that is required by a medical practitioner.

Author though followed Madhavanidana and brihatrayee to a larger extent in compiling the text but he was not hesitant to unfollow them, thus he deviated many a time with reference to classification of diseases, separate chapters have been allocated for sannipata prkaranam, ksaya prakaranam and sopha prakaranam because he consideres them as important. He identifies many new clinical conditions and also prepared many new formulations to his credit.

In kshaya prakaranam author gives peculiar description about the disease Ksaya.In it we find unique description about the kingdom of ksaya roga in which jwara is the king, kamila is his wife, panduroga is the general of the army and Raktapittam (bleeding disorder) as his (syndromes) son etc.

क्षयरोगे ज्वरो राजा तस्य पत्नितु कामिल

चमुपतिहि पाण्डुरोगो रक्तपित्तस्य पुत्रक: chapter5/1

Author could identify certain group of medical conditions like Mahakshaya, pandukshaya, ajirna kshaya and depicted them as serious debilitating and incurable. The above said clinical conditions could well be correlated with cachexia of several malignancies and auto immune disorders.

His clinical expertise in the preparations of the formulations can be understood by the selection of drugs for bhavana and mardana . It is evident in the preparation of formulations he used highest number of bhavana dravya, prakshepa dravya to get the desired pharmacological effect in a given disease. And, he administered these formulations in many different diseases with mere change of anupana.

For example Lokanatharasa a formulation mentioned in ksaya prakaranam is administered in various diseases with mere change of anupana.

Eg., In jwara Lokanatharasa administered along with dhanyaka and guduchi kashaya, and in Atisara with dadima swarasa etc.

Many times his formulations named according to the treating disease (Eg., nisa jwara kashaya, sandhya jwara kashaya of jwara prakaranam or the name of the formulation depended on the main drug used in the formulations or the name indicated of the rishi who formulated it. eg Parasara ghrtam (formulated by acharya Parasara).

Vallabhacharya is specific about the time administration of medicine.

Eg., Maha soubhaya shunti advised to be administered in pratahakala (early morning).

Ayurvedic formulations mostly prepared according to putapaka vidhi (churna mixed with ghrta and kept under eranda patra and made into pottali and heated on mandagni and processed) and by rasakriya (churna prepared into kashaya $1/4^{th}$ of it and with other drugs and cooked into avalehapaka. After having cooled, appropriate quantity of madhu is added and administered).

In Vaidya chintamani we find liberal use of bhang (cannabis sativa) in the formulations. We see bhang as ingredient for many of the preparations like Lahi churna (sangrahani roga) . In this formulation Bhang is added ½ of the quantity of total drugs added. In jatiphaladi churnam a formulation mentioned in kshaya prakaranam we find bhang is used in highest quantity (386grams) . And also, even use of bhang mentioned in sangrahani while mentioning of pathya . In sigrupushpa rasayanam (Prameha), jatyadi vati etc., formulations of prameha bhang is added 4 parts.

In the treatment of sangrahani, ahiphena administered to cure atisara and in painful conditions .

Eg., Daradadi putapaka, and jatiphaladi putapaka .

In the formulation of Grahani gaja keasri rasa we observe that 5 parts of ahiphena is added while other drugs added 1 part each to cure raktaja grahani associated with pain. In some of the yogas ahiphena added 7 parts and abhraka added 25 parts. It appears he has excellent knowledge about each of the drug and basing on it he used a particular drug which he considers best added in abundance to get the desired effect in a given clinical condition.

The peculiarity of Madhu pakvva haritaki formulation is that in this Haritaki is taken 100 in number and heated in dolayantra process. After they got cooked properly, haritaki are punctured and collected in a container, to this container 100 pala of madhu is added, with this haritaki looses its kashaya taste then fine powder of pippali etc drugs are added to it before administration.

Describing Agnikumararasa a formulation of vata prakaranam, author mentions that if agnikumararasa is administered on head (siras) by piercing with needle cures sannipata condition (critical condition) to make the patient alive.

Formulation Vyaghri taila mentioned in Vata prakaranam contains spurious liquor ½ part and pravata mrittika (soil collected from mountains) as their ingredients.

Durva ghrtam (Raktapitta prakaranam) is administered as vasti in the conditions of bleeding from penis and also in bleeding per rectum. In the conditions of bleeding from roots of hairs, application of this ghrta is advised.

Maha cincadi lehyam a formulation of pitta prakaranam contains 109 drugs in which we find 35 prakshepa dravya added.

In the preparation of Kankayana gutika we observe increasing pattern of the quantity of ingredients such as pippalee, pippalee mulam, chitrakam, sonthi, yavaksharam taken in the order 1, 2, 3, 4, 5, 6, 7, 8 palas respectively.

In Hikka prakaranam a formulation namely Makshika sakritasya is prepared from makshika vista (sediment of of honey) or laksa (laccifer lacca), candana triturated in sthanya and administered as nasya for the treatment of Hikka.

In the preparations of dhupa we find weird syubstances like dung of deer, dung of wild pig feather of peacock, sarpa kurpasa (external skin layer of snake) tail, sting of scorpion, wings of dragon fly are used (Eg.kshetra palika dhupa of sannipata prakaranam) .

While mentioning of apathya of Arsa roga kathina kukkutasana contra indicated. Thus it can be deducted that in those days every day yoga was a common practice.

In the preparations of lepa (external applications), we find the ingredients like bhallataka (semecarpus anacardium), tusk of elephant. Shit of pigeon vatsanabhi, arsenic oxide (gauri pashana) etc., are used.

In krimi roga, a formulation (bahya krmi lepa) consists of mercury (parada). It is given mardana in Krishna dattura patra swarasa and thus obtained paste is pasted over cloth and then this cloth is applied over the head for 3 yama then the yuka present in the head will die and get attached to the cloth.

Author many a time either added slokas or deleted certain slokas in a chapter taken from the books like madhava nidana etc. (eg., sloka depicting the use of trikatu churna in adhogata amlapitta) .And also, we see such changes made in mahakhandhardrakam of amlapitta. Generally Ayurveda scholars (authors) do not consider it proper of such deletion or adding of stanzas or verses to the verses taken from the original texts of Ayurveda.

In those days it appears that there is a regular practice of performing homa and other vrata, japa etc (daivavyapasraya chikitsa) as a measure of prayaschitta to get rid from the bad effects of karmavipaka, astrological abnormalities of the person.

In the book Vaidyacintamani different varieties of mandura are mentioned in Panduprakaranam .We observe that in one of the preparation of mandura vataka (panduroga) urine of different animals were used like gomutra, ajamutra, beda mutra (urine of sheep), ustramutra, gardabhamutra, hastimutra and asvamutra.

In the preparations of lepa (External applications) stree stanya (breast milk) also added as an ingredient (sannipata prakaranam).

It appears that it is a regular practice in the preparations of formulations adding up with clinically proven churna (drug powder) in abundance to kashayas (decoctions) probably to potentiate the medicine. Eg., In swasa prakaranam pippali churnam added with drakshadi kashaya, puskaramula churna added with the kuluthadi kashaya. It is observed that many a time pippali churna mixed with kashaya commonly.

In pitta prakaranam he mentions about 24 varieties of pittaroga such classification is not available in any other text. Eg., avarana paitya, vivarna paitya, amla paitya etc., many a time author deviates from main Ayurveda texts and presents his own dictum.

In kshaya prakaranam talaka sindura (prepared from suddha haratala and suddha manshila) is administered in different diseases with change of swarasa and churna. Eg., Talakasindura administered with gokshura swarasa in raktapitta, talak sindura administered with haritaki churna in swasa, and with pippalichurna in kasa. It appears that selecting of churna is based on his clinical experience, amazingly his thoughts coinside with present modern clinical research.

In some of the preparations we observe the pattern of adding drug in the ascending order.Eg., in Karpuradi churnam of aruci prakaranam drugs like karpura12gm, lavanga, 24 gram nagakesara 36 gm added in ascending order.

Author advocates even what kind of mrttika is to be used in the formulations. Many a time he mentions about saurashtra mrittika . (mud of saurashtra (a place around Gujarat) .

In sula prakaranam, an external application over the umbilicus mentioned to relieve from colic. Rajika (brassica juncea) and sigru (moringa) are to be triturated in gotakra (cow's butter milk) and thus prepared lepa is to be applied on umbilicus.

Author widely uses lavanas and kshara such as saindhava, samudra, vida, samudra lavana, sauvarcala lavana and arka snuhi, cincha sarja yava kshara, sura kshara, snuhi kshara in the formulations respectively. Eg., sankha vatika (gulma prakaranam) .

Pancakarma is not mentioned as a separate entity in the treatment of individual diseases.

We also find indication of gomutra pana added with vidanga and kustha in the treatment krimija hridroga.

In hridroga we find a formulation prepared with dugdhapan (24 pala) added wih sita and honey. The important formulation by him is nagabaladi dugdhapana.

We find references of exclusive administration of rasabhasma (mercury), Tamra bhasma and gandhaka as follows. Rasabhasma administered with madhu, tamra bhasma added with pippali curna and suddha gandhaka added with adhuka taila in the tretmant of medoroga .

We find a formulation (visuci kasaya) in which urine of child boy is collected and boiled and added with pippali churna and administered. Other scholars opine that it should be read as bala mulasya (mulaka which is not ripen).

In upadamsa roga (veneral disease) several types of prakshalana drava (cleaning liquids) like aswathadi, jayadi prakshalana are described. These are disinfectant decoctions used to clean the wound.

In mukha roga, formulations like lakshadi taila to strengthen the gums mentioned. Preparation of tooth powder is mentioned i.e., kustadi churna a formulation comprising of kusta, katuk, haridra prepared into powder for this purpose .We see the practice of Jati patradi curna kept in the mouth to get rid of inflammation of ulcers of the mouth.

In mukha roga prakaranam we find the reference of galasundika chedan vidhi (incision).

Among karna roga (ear diseases) there is mention of putikarna (ear discharge), for which special formulations like Dipika yoga are mentioned. Varti prepared from brihat panchamula immersed in tila taila and the stem is burnt Taila falling in drops are collected and this taila in lukewarm state used as ear drops. There is mention about krimi karna (ear infested by worms) and putikarna. Amradi taila and gandhaka taila exclusively prepared for the treatment of chronic ulcer with sinus of ear. Chitraka haritaki rasayana administered in sosa (cachexia), pratisyaya (coryza) . We find treatment for polyps of the nose with griha dhuma taila etc.

Preparations of Kanadi nasya, vyaghri taila are exclusively indicated for puti nasya (suppurative nasal discharge).

Description of Siro roga and its varities are mentioned as 11. They are vata, pitta, kapha, sannipata, raktaja, kshyaja, krimija, anantavata, ardhavabhedaka, and sankhaka.

Formulations mentioned for these sirorogas are Navanatha siddha taila, tiktakosataki taila, sadbindu taila gained popularity. Author elaborately discusses about causes for eye diseases. He explains that the eye diseases are 94. He describes 8types abhishyanda (conjunctivitis), adhimantha (glaucoma), timira roga, linganasa (cataract) pothaki etc., important diseases have been mentioned. Several anjanas like trikatukadyanjana, garudadyanjana, mahanarikelanjana, pushpanjana, chandrodaya varti etc mentioned.

Under the chapter suddhiprakaranam we find sodhana of sapta loha i.e swarna, rajata, tamra, pittala, naga, vanga and tikshna loha. He explains dhatu sodhana, bhasma vidhi, and its disease indication along with anupana for each one of the dhatu.

Elaborate description about parada (mercury) is available. Purification of Parada is mentioned as mandatory before its administration hence describes procedures for removing its astadosa. There is description of astadasa samskaras of parada, pathya and apathya during rasaushadhi sevana is explained. A detailed explanation is given about rasakarpura, gandhaka, abhraka (biotite Mica), haratala (orpiment) and anjana to improve the eye sight. Kasisa (green vitriol), gairika (red ochre), Hingula (cinnabar), manashila (realgar) sankha (conch) described. later he describes about origin of upadhatu. eg swarna makshika is upadahatu of swarna.

We get description about girisindhura (red oxide of mercury), gauripashana (arsenic oxide), silajitu (mineral pitch) kampilla, mastaki, Kharpar is given. We get detailed description about sarjaksharam, yavakshara (potassium salts), pancalavana, trikatu and vatsanabha, and also about their sodhana.

Later we get descriptions about navaratna, vajra (diamond), mukta (pearl), vaikrannta etc. lastly he describes about kritrima Visa (artificial poison), visa of scorpion, and snake bites and its treatments.

In yantra prakaranam we find description of yantras. These yantras are specially designed equipemnnt used for preparation of medicines out of metals etc.These equipements can be preared by clay, iron or stainless steel. He describes about vidhyadhara yantra, tanka yantra, valuka yantra, garbha yantra jala yantra, gauri yantra, bhudhara yantra, kosti yantra, tula yantra, dola yantra, patala yantra and Tejo yantra.

Author mentions about verities of puta like mahaputa, varahaputa kapota puta, etc,

In manaprakaranam, he describes about weights and measurements .In this chapter description about Magadha prastha and standardization about prastha according to Bhojaraja and also sadharana tulamana (measurements) are given. Descriptions about various measurements like paramanu, marici, rajika, yava, gunja, masa, kola, karsa pala etc available in the book.

Under Paribhasa prakaranam he explains about the technical terms mentioned in sastra.

Among plants some plant roots, in some plants bark etc is useful in the preparation of formulatons. Author categorizes and describes them as kandasara (best in rhizomes or roots

), mulasara (best in roots), mulatwaksara (best in root bark), darutwak sar (the bark of stem) sara sara (heartwood), patrasara, puspasara phala sara (fruits) bijasara etc are given.This information useful because cetain part of the pant works better when compared to other parts in a given disease . We get information about alabdha pratinidhi dravya. If there is no information about which part of plant to be used in a given disease, author gives some clues for it. When a part of the plant not specified then the root of the plant to be used if that is not also availble similar root to be used as pratinidhi dravya (substitute of drugs) i.e when a particular drug is not available almost a suitable drug is being mentioned by the author .

Later he gives classification of drugs set as a group having same properties and therapeutic action.Eg., dasamula, pancakola (pippali, pippalimula, cavya, chitraka and nagara are the group of drugs called as panchakola) .

In the book Vaidyacintamani women and children diseases are not mentioned. And also, Rasayana and vajikarana too have not mentioned. Many new clinical disorders are mentioned in Vaidyacintamani and we find mentions of these clinical conditions in the subsequent texts like Basavarajiya, Vaidyayogaratnavali etc.

Mostly author of Vaidyacintamani has taken verses from books like Madhavanidana and Madhava kalpa, however, author did not mention about the source from where he has taken the verses. Number of authors referred to Vaidyacintamani but it is difficult for us to know which is the original since many authors having the same book title as vaidya chintamani.

It is interesting to note that while mentioning about disease kshaya, all types of kshaya result due to the sin of killing of woman in previous birth. And also, it is amazing to note that the person will have several births. It is surprising to note that on which number of birth, at what age of the patient, what type of kshaya will occur. Likewise there is description of the origin of 20 kshaya, namely Raktakshaya, Rajayakshma, santapakshaya, murchakshaya, soshakshaya, vamanakshaya, grahanee shulakshaya, sophakshaya, suskashaya, Atisarakshaya mandagnikshaya, vivarnakshaya, ajeernakshaya, tiktakshaya udgara, kshaya dahakshaya, tandrakshaya, kshaya, darunakshaya, haridrakshaya respectively.

eg., In the 1st birth At 5 years of age one will develop rakta kshaya.

Each of the twenty varieties of kshaya is explained with specific characteristics . for example in Rakta Kshaya the specific features are as follows. If Kshaya exists for more than eight, ten, fifteen, one month, two months or six months and bleeds from nose, mouth, rectum, ears and suffers from weakness, loss of appetite, cough and sputum considered as Rakta Kshaya. Likewise the important features for all the kshayas are explained.

Another important contributing feature is mentioning of survival period for each of the Kshaya .For example the patient of Rakta Kshaya will suffer for 5 months. Likewise, author has given suffering period for all types of kshaya is amazing. It is surprising to note that they were in a position to identify a given clinical condition as a separate clinical entity inspite of having similar symptoms in many of the diseases.

It is mentioned that disease itself as a causative factor for other disease in Vaidyachintamani .Eg Jwara Santapa cause raktapitta. In modern parlance psoriasis causes arthritis can be taken as analogy.

Many terms belonging to telugu (a language spoken by andhrapradesh of southern india) Like goranta (henna), vanti (vomiting), malabaddhata (constipation), maha nissattuva etc., hence it can be presumed that the author belongs to Andhra desa.

Doshatisara lakshana a separate clinica condition mentioned in atisara prakaranam. We see use of the term gudaroga (probably indicating of piles and fistula) in atisara (diarrhea and dysentery) prakaranam.

We find extensive descriptions about mandura (iron based medicine) and its varieties mainly administered in panduroga.

Contrary to main texts of Ayurveda like caraka, susruta and vagbhata he gives a separate classification to certain diseases. In Sopha (odema or swelling) prakaranam, we observe a different classification like pasana sopha (swelling due to arsenic poisioning), vrana jwara sopha, kadgaghata sopha, kamila sopha (Swelling due to jaundice), gandhaka sopha (allergic inflammation due to sulphur) etc are mentioned.

Chapter on Madatyaya mostly taken from Madhavanidana but number of stanzas deleted from it. Added verse state that proper amount of madya to be drunk for rasayana (rejuvenation) purpose.

Aditional verses are added to verses while describing about pathogenesis of masurika, sital stotra japa, maharudra, eight measures to cure jwara, krsihnasmarana etc.

Added verses of kusta roga depict about the incurability of some kusta.

We find added verses on sthana vidradhi, upadamsa, pitta rakta, vatarakta and kshudraroga . Additional stanzas are given on mukharoga, nasarogas, nasarsas, pinasa, karnataravrana, netra rogas. Types of disease enumeration differ from main ayurvedic texts.

In those days there is a practice of worshipping an idol which used to represent each disease. Each idol differs with each of the disease.The patient suffering from kamala should perform puja to statue of atanka devata possessing yellow coloured body, skull in one hand and musalayudham in other hand.

In kamila prakaranam the formulation punaranavadi leha highest number of prakshepa dravya (Fine powder form of the drug (s) added to Leha, Āsavāriṣṭa etc. before administration.

In kshaya prakaranam under the formulation Navaratna raja mriganka rasa we find highest number of bhavana dravya.

Just as brihatrayee in Vaidyacintamani too there is mention of signs and symptoms indicating incurability (asadhya lakshana) for every disease. Eg., At the end of sannipata jwara severe swelling occur over the root of the ear is considered as asdhya lakshana.In pandu, swelling of akshikuta (surrounding of he veye, ganda (cheeks), bru (forehead, pada, nabhi, medhra (penis) is considered as asadhya.

Sopha (oedema) occurring in the middle portion of the body, sopha which is spread in all parts of the body considered as asadhya. In Atisara if a person passess stools similar to colour of ripened black berry jamun fruit, similar to colour of liver or mutton wash water or mala (stool) similar to curd, oil, or ghee considered as asadhya, likewise we get number of asadhya lakshanas mentioned for each of the disease.

TABLE OF CONTENTS

CONCEPT OF KARMA VIPAKA 1

JYOTISSASTRABHIPRAYAM (ASTROLOGICAL CONSIDERATIONS) AS A CAUSATION OF DISEASE 34

ASHTA STHANA PARIKSHA 38

SALIENT FEATURES OF DISEASES MENTIONED IN VAIDYACINTAMANI 50

VISHA PRAKARANAM 141

SUDDHIPRAKARANAM 146

YANTRA PRAKARANAM 194

MANA PRAKARANAM (WEIGHTS AND MEASUREMENTS) 206

PARIBHASA PARAKARANAM 210

AMAZING PRESCRIPTIONS, METHODS OF PREPARATIONS AND ADMINISTERING METHODS 215

ANUPANAS MENTIONED IN VAIDYACINTAMANI 236

PATHYA AND APATHYA OF DISEASES 245

NAMES OF RISHIS WHO HAVE FORMULATED AND PROPAGATED A GIVEN YOGA. 250

FREQUENTLY USED DRUGS IN VAIDYACHINTAMANI 251

ANNEXURE 1: 263

APPENDIX 281

CONCEPT OF KARMA VIPAKA

Author mentions that karmavipaka (sin of previous birth) as a causative factor for the disease.for almost all the diseses karmavipaka is mentioned. He explains pacifying measures such as daivavyapasraya chikitsa along with internal medication for it. This kind of concept stating karma vipaka as the causative factor for the disease is unique of him.

Notes: *The concept of karma vipaka appears to be new contribution by the author and is as follows.The diseases we suffer from the births we get here on earth are all products of actions done by us in previous times. Every action has its reaction and no action goes unrewarded in a suitable manner. Evil actions do not go without their bitter effects upon the doer. Probably this concept is more prevalent during Vallabhendra period.*

Daiva vyapasraya chikitsa is the treatment for diseases arising due to purva janmakruta papa karma (sins of past life) or karmaja vyadhis (karmic ailments) . This type of treatment was done in the Rigvedic period in majority and yuktivyapasharaya was neglected. The observance of yama (ahimsa (non violence), satya (truth), astaya (not to steal), bramhacharya (control over sexual desire), and aparigraha (accumulation of prosperities)) and niyama (shaucha (cleanliness), santosha (satisfaction), tapas (conquest of all desires), swadhyaya (self-study), ishwara pranidhana (surrender to God)) is also part of this treatment. This form of treatment includes chanting mantras, wearing amulets on body, wearing gems, precious stones etc. performing auspicious rituals, offerings to God, oblations, homa, following niyama, prayachhitta, upavasa, svastyayana, pranipata and going to holy places.

The following are the karma vipaka mentioned for each disease along with their pacifying measures.

In Jwara prakaranam author explaining Karma Vipaka of jwara states that stealing of deva dravya as the sole cause for the causation of fevers. While describing about seetajwara he explains that it occurs in those who indulge in Krura Karma (Cruel acts), sinful acts and back biting.

देवस्वहरणाच्चैव जायते विविधो ज्वरः ।
ज्वरो महाज्वरश्चैव रौद्रो वैष्णव एव च ।। ३ ।।

Notes: *Jwara is an important disease. The term 'Jwara' implies the ability of a disease to cause anguish to body and mind. This suggests suffering or illness. Based on the similarity in clinical features, Jwara is often considered as fever or pyrexia in medical terminologies. However, according to Ayurveda, the classical description of jwara includes variety of other clinical conditions with or without rise in body temperature. Therefore, fever or hyperpyrexia is considered as only one among the many features of jwara.*

Author mentioning Kshayaroga Karma Vipaka that it occurs in persons who murders brahmana and who usurps the land of brahmana or murders a woman. The persons without having the knowledge of traditional religious laws if punishes others will suffer from kshaya.

Who suffers from kshaya, as a penance should make a golden banana tree with leaves and fruits .He has to tie a cloth and thread to it and perform puja (prayer) .He should also provide delicious food to brahmana and request him to undertake homa. After Homa, the patient should donate the golden banana tree by chanting hiranya garbha purusha mantra to him so as to get relieved from kshaya (pthisis) disease.

There is also mention of Ksaya rogahara pratima danam. In order to pacify the sin, he has to donate a statue designed as follows. It should have dhanus (bow) with an arrow about to be released in the hand and the forefinger of the right hand to frighten and should have three eyes. It should bite its lower lips with upper sharp teeth and should ready to kill the bad elements. The person to get rid of disease should follow brahmacharya, giving donations, should perform tapas and puja following traditions and truth. He should also perform surya namaskaras, vaidya puja and brahmana puja.

Notes:

The term kshaya refers to decrease or depletion of body tissues and also of tridosha. Here author refers to the disease similar to Rajayakshma mentioned in brihatrayee for kshaya. Rajayakshma is a syndrome consisting of diseases associated with wasting (kshaya) of various tissues including rasa and ojas causing immunodeficiency. The term rajayakshma has been used interchangeably with tuberculosis. It is potentially fatal wasting disease that "consumes" the body.

Panduroga: देवद्विज द्रव्यहारी पांडुरोगी भवेन्नरः । कृच्छ्यातिकृच्छ्रो कुर्याच्च चांद्रायणमतंद्रितः ॥ ३॥ कुर्यात्कूश्मांड होमं च स्वर्ण चंद्रेण वाससी । ब्राह्मणेभ्यो यथाशक्ति दद्यात् पांडु निवृत्तये ॥४॥

Describing Karma Vipaka of panduroga author states that the disease results because of robbing or stealing of deva brahmana dravya. To pacify this one should perform prayaschitta by performing difficult procedure of candrayana vrata and kushmanda homa then donate idol of chandrama made up of gold and cloths to brhmana according to his capacity to get relieved from panduroga. Pandu roga (resembling with anemia) is characterized by pallor which is associated with different colors according to dosha involved. Aggravated pitta predominant dosha vitiates the dhatu. This vitiation of dhatu cause sluggishnesss (shithilata) and heaviness (gaurava) in the dhatu resulting in diminution of complexion (varna), strength (bala), unctuousness (sneha) and the qualities of ojas. Thus, the person develops diminished blood (rakta) and the fatty tissue (meda dhatu) and absence of the vitality of all the tissues (nihsara) decreases functional Status of sense organs (sithilendryah) and cause discouloration of the body. Author also describing karma vipaka of siroroga sahita pandu (Anaemia associated with disorders of the head) says that it affects such persons who initiate but do not complete the procedure agnistomadi karma. Such affected people as a measure of penance must perform krichra, atikrichra and chandrayana vrata and also provide sumptuous meal to hundred brahmana to get rid of the disease.

Kamala:

Notes: *Kamala is the term used in Ayurveda to describe a disease, which resembles Jaundice. Pandu and Kamala are said to be the diseases, which are interrelated. A person with jaundice may notice a yellowish tinge to their skin, mucous membranes, and the whites of the eyes. It can happen with various health conditions and usually indicates a problem with the liver or bile ducts.*

Explaining Karma Vipaka of Kamala author writes that the person who steals rice (anna) will be affected with the disease kamala. As a measure of penance to get rid of the disease kamala an effigy of Garutmanta to be prepared with gold who bears Lord Mahavishnu on his back, the size of idol prepared depending on ones own financial capability. The idol should consist of two pearls and a diamond to adorn wings and the nose respectively.

पीतांगः कामिला रोगः कपालमुसलान्वितः ॥ ५ ॥

पूजाविधाने त्वातंक देवतात्व उदाहतः

The patient of kamala has to prepare an idol of diety named as "atanka devata". This idol of diety should hold the weapon (musala yudha) and skull in the hand made up of gold, and this should be donated to as per the norms of "Atanka Vidhi" .The idol should be wrapped with white cloth yarned with silver. Rupee coins should be kept in ghrita droni and is worshipped with white flowers. After this, a pious Brahmin who is well versed with all sastra, and also a devotee of Vishnu should be worshipped with sodashopachara then the idol should be donated.

Atisara:

Notes: *Diarrhoea is described in Ayurvedic classics with the name of "Atisara". It means excessive flow of watery stool through anus. It is resulted due to jataragni mandhya (low digestive fire) . Weak digestive fire, improper food, impure water, toxins and mental stress usually cause atisaram.*

Karma Vipaka of Atisara mentions that brahmin who leaves smartagni will get affected with Atisara. To get rid of this one should chant a ruk known as "agnirasmi" and from that one tenth part Ajyasahita tila should be given in homa.

One who destroys tretagni will get atisara. He should prepare the statue of bright agni sitting on a sheep (akuljwala) with 1pala or ½ pala of gold or copper as per his capacity pasted with raktachandana, it is decorated with rakta vastra and adorned with redcolour garland, pearl chains which shine equal to meru parvata and dwadasaarka (12 suns) and it is donated to agnihotri brahmacari brahmana along with clothes chanting below mentioned mantra.

In Atisara Prakarana author explains dana mantra (chanting of mantra while donating) .

त्रेताऽरूपोग्निरीड्यस्त्वंमं ततश्चासि वै नृणाम् ।। ८ ।।

त्वं वेत्थ प्राक्तनं पापमतिसारं विनाशया । एवं कृत्वा नरः सम्यगतिसारं व्यपोहति । नीरुजः स सुखी नित्यं दीर्घमायुः स विंदति ।

It states that "O" agni you are in three ways (garhapatya, havaneya and daksinagni) .one which engulfs the humans at the end, and the one who knows the good and sins of previous births of the human beings, may get rid of this disease atisara". The person who donates while chanting the above said mantra not only gets freed from atisara but also lives for hundred years in happiness without disease.

The person who kills woman in previous birth gets affected with the disease atisara. To repel the disease ten aswatha (peepal trees) are to be planted and should donate dhenu with sarkara and also to provide meal to hundred brahmana.

Grahani:

Notes :

Grahani is an ayurveda term related to the seat of agni (digestive fire), which help in the metabolism and digestion of food. The ancient text of ayurveda described that ingestion, digestion, absorption and assimilation of Aahaar is regulated by Grahani. When this Agni becomes manda then improper digestion of ingested food leads pathological condition termed as Grahani roga. Similarly three types anomalies of the Jatharagni also termed as Grahanidosha.

अनन्य गतिकां भार्यमिदुष्टां कारणं विना । परित्यजति यः स्सोऽपि ग्रहणीरोगवान् भवेत् ॥ शिवसंकल्प सूक्तस्य जपः स्यात्तत्र शान्तये । अष्टोत्तरसहस्रं हि हिरण्यं च तथा मधु ॥२॥ दद्याद्वित्तानुसारेण सौरमंत्रं जपेत्तथा । धेनुं सलक्षणां दद्याद्रत्नाभरणसंयुताम् ॥३॥ पयस्विनीं गुणोपेतां ब्राह्मणाय कुटुंबिने । वत्साभरणसंयुक्तच ॥४॥ (grahani)

Author explaining karmavipaka of Grahani says that the one who abandons wife for no reason though she is loyal and polite to him will be afflicted by the disease grahani.

As a penance one should chant siva sukta one thousand eight times and also donate gold and honey by chanting souramantra. After that he has to donate a cow along with its calf possessing good qualities and gives lots of milk and after it being decorated with clothes and ornaments to a married brahmin after the Brahmin also being adorned with clothes and ornaments.

Gudaroga: Author states that the person who abuses temples and also water will suffer from dreadful disease gudaroga (disease related to rectum).

सुरालये जले वापि शकृद्दोषं करोति यः । गुदरोगो भवेत्तस्य पापरूपः सुदारुणः ॥ ५ ॥ मासं सुरार्चनेनैव गोदानद्वितयेन च । प्राजापत्येन चैकेन शाम्यंति गुदजा रुजः ॥ ६ ॥

As a part of penance he must worship the diety for one month and also should donate cows two in number or perform praja pathya krichram.

Notes:

The term gudaroga derived from local language telugu since he belonged to Andhradesa i.e Andhrapradesh. Probably the term comprises the diseases piles, fistula, tumors of rectum.

Vatavyadhi: Explaining Karmavipaka of vatavyadhi author writes that the one who in his previous birth steals or robs money of brahmanas or devata or the one who betrays the master gets affected with vata disease. To get relieve from vata he has to make expiation (prayaschittam).

A person who hates his teacher will get vata disease. The person should perform sacrifice (homas) by chanting.

To repel and pacify karma vipaka one should perform Japa (muttering of prayers) by chanting Achyuta, Ananta and govinda nama.

Notes:

Vatavyadhi Chikitsa deals with diseases particularly caused by vata dosha. It is an important chapter as it encompasses a large spectrum of disorders especially concerned with neurological system, musculoskeletal system, reticulo-endothelial system and further pervades to all other systems in the body.

Dhanurvata: Explaining Karmavipaka of Dhanurvata author writes that the one who indulges in sex with woman by force suffers from Dhanurvata associated with severe pain in all over the joints, loss of taste, and fever.

अनिच्छदक्षतां यस्तु ह्युपभुंक्ते परस्त्रियम् । बलादाक्रम्य स नरःसर्व संधिषु वेदनाम् ॥४॥ तीव्रामाप्नोत्यरुचिमान्धनुर्वातयुतो भवेत् । ज्वरी तदुपशांत्यर्थं महिषीदानमाचरेत् ॥ ५ ॥ कृच्छ्रतिकृच्छ्रौ कुर्वीत चांद्रायणमथापरम् । सूर्यनाम जपं चैव शक्त्या ब्राह्मणतर्पणम् ॥ ६ ॥ नामत्रयं जपेन्मर्त्यो रोगशान्त्यर्थमात्मनः । सहस्रनामकं चापि स्तोत्रं सम्यग्विधानतः ॥७॥ अच्युतानंतगोविंदेत्येतन्नामत्रयं द्विजः । अयुत्रितया वृत्त्या जपेद्रोगस्य शांतये ॥ ८ ॥

To repel this the affected should donate buffalo and should perform krichram, atikrichram, chandrayana, should chant soura mantra and provide meal to brahmana. The affected should mutter names of Achyuta, Ananta, govinda and sahasra nama stotra (chanting of thousand names of dieties) and also parayana (reading a holy book regularly) is to be undertaken.

Notes:

Dhanurvata or Dandaka is described under Vatavyadhi similar to Tetanus. Tetanus is a serious disease caused by bacteria that affects the nervous system and causes the tightening of the whole muscle in the infected host. It is also referred to as lockjaw because it tightens the muscle of the neck and jaws and sometime body curves like bow hence known as dhanurvata in Ayurveda .

Pakshaghata:

सभायां पक्षपाती च जायते पक्षघातवान् । निष्कत्रयमितं हेम स दद्याच्च द्विजातये ॥ ९ ॥ श्राद्धं च वैष्णवं कुर्यादात्मनो हितमिच्छता । सप्तधान्यानि दद्याच्च गोदानं चापि कारयेत् ॥ १० ॥

Author explaining Karmavipaka of Pakshaghata that who speaks with prejudice and bias supporting a particular group in meetings will get pakshghata. To repel this gold weighing 3 niska pramana has to be donated to a brahmin and also he should perform vaishnava srartha and saptadhanya dana and also he has to donate a cow.

Notes:

Paralysis in Ayurveda is called as Pakshaghata which is one of the Vata vyadhis mentioned in the classical texts. Paralysis is characterized by a loss of muscle strength and functioning in a part of the body. This is primarily due to a problem with the nerve connections between the brain and the affected body part which result in a loss of muscle strength and movement.

Raktavata: Author explaining Karmavipaka of Rakta vata mentions that the person who steals red clothes, coral will get the disease rakta vata. As a penance, one should donate she buffalo along with rubies (padmaraga) and a red cloth to a Brahmin.

Notes:

The disease Raktavata not mentioned as separate entity as disease.In Ayurvedic texts we find references as rakta gata vata and vatarakta. This is coined term by the author and the symptoms of raktavata are having the close resemblance with the disease vatarakta.

Vatarakta and vatapitta:

सवर्णागमने वातरक्तवाज्ञायते

वातरक्तवाज्ञायते नरः । असवर्णागमे वातपित्तवानपि जायते ॥१२॥
लक्ष्मीनारायणं रूपं सुवर्णेन प्रकल्पयेत् । पलेन वा तदर्धेन तदर्धेनाथवा ददेत्
॥१३॥ लक्ष्मीनारायणरूपं सर्वदा सर्वदा सर्वकामदम्

Author explaining Karmavipaka of Vatarakta and Vatapitta mentions that The one who indulges is sex with woman of same gotra will get vatarakta disease. or the one who indulges sex other than his wife belongs to other caste will be afflicted by the disease vata pitta. To pacify this an idol of lakshminarayana prepared from gold weighing pala, a half pala or ¼ pala should be donated to Brahmana. The one who consumes garlic, bhang and tatiphala (fruit of palymra tree) will be affected by the disease vata pitta. To repel this, thay should perform chandrayana vrata.

Notes:

Vatarakta as the name suggest is the vitiation of Vata Dosha and Rakta Dhatu (blood) . In this condition the normal flow of Vata is obstructed by Rakta leading to symptoms starting from Paada (foot) and Hasta (hands) causing pain in them. This disease similar to Gout. Gout occurs when urate crystals accumulate in joint, causing the inflammation and intense pain of a gout attack. Urate crystals can form when high levels of uric acid in the blood. Vatapitta is aggravation of vata and pitta. In a disease but in brihatrayee we do not find vatapittaas a separate disease

Raktapitta:

मद्यपो रक्तपित्तीस्यात्स दद्यात्सर्पिषो घटम् । मधुनोऽर्धघटं चैव सा हिरण्यं विशुद्धये ॥ १ ॥

चंद्रक्षेत्रे यदा भौमो जायते मुनजस्तदा । रक्तपित्ती च दुर्नाम नानाव्याधिसमाकुलः ॥२॥ रक्तपित्तं ज्वरं दाहमग्निवयवोरुपद्रवम् । लभते नात्र संदेहश्चंद्रमध्ये यदा कुजः ॥३॥ भौममंत्रजपः कार्यो होमः खादिरजैः तिलैः । घृतेन च समायुक्तैर्दानं रक्तवृषस्य च ॥४॥ बिल्वचंदनबलाशाणपुष्पैरिंगुदीकफलिनीवकुलैश्च ।

स्नानमद्भिरिहमग्नियुताभिर्भीमदोष विनिवारणमाशु ॥५॥

Author explaining Karmavipaka of Raktapitta describes that the person who consumes alcohol in his previous birth will be afflicted by the disease rakta pitta. In order to get rid of the disease such patient should donate a pot full of ghee and half potful of honey along with gold to get relieved from the disease.

Notes :

Raktapitta is a bleeding disorder where in the blood (Rakta) vitiated by Pitta flows out of the orifices (openings) of the body.

Aruchi, shula & chardhi:

Author explaining Karmavipaka of aruchi, shula & chardi states that in order to get rid of the disorder expiations of krichra, atikrichra, chandrayana have to be performed depending on the gradation of the disease. The person who experiences inability of performing the above said prayascita, and if he is rich enough should provide sumptuous meal to fifty brahmanas. If the patient is poor, then he should resort to Japa, homa, teerthasnana, developing and deep philosophical attitude and also providing meal to brahmana to the extent possible by him to get relieved by the disease.

Person who with perverted mind deliberately provides polluted food with hair, insects and the food touched with crows and dogs, and also the one who betrays will develop the disease chardhi. To repel this, annadana should be performed to brahmana along with ghee.

Notes:

A condition of the Lack of desire to eat principal meals or break fast is called Arochaka . Shoola can be considered as colicky type of pain in the abdomen. Vomiting is described as forceful expulsion of contents of stomach through mouth and sometimes nose. The term Chardi can be correlated with vomiting or emesis in modern medicine.

Kasa : Author explaining of karmavipaka of kasa mentions that the person who steels by cheeting from poor people, then he will get kapha disease leading to kasa (cough), and also he should perform santapana krichra to get relieved from kasa.

According to other the personwho steels trapu (tin) then he will suffer from kapha disease.To get rid of it he has to stay without food for one day and the next day he has to donate trapu weighing 400 tolas.

As per another version yama deva told that a man who leaves regular costumes then he will suffer from kapha, gets defeated by enemies.To get relieve from kasa he has to eat yavakannam for one month and he has to perform a sacrifice (homa) with chervajya dravyas for 1008 times along with chanting Vishnu sahasranama.

Swasa:

Author explaining Karmavipaka of Swasa etc., mentions that the person who is ungrateful will get the disease kapha, swasa, kasa, usna Jwara and pittaroga. To repel he has to perform expiations of three chandrayana Krichra, and also should provide meals to fifty Brahmins. He should also chant Vishnusahasranama japa and worship devabrahmana with utmost respect.

Others opinion of karmavipaka is that the person who receives donations like mahadana or nishiddhadana at the time of grahanadi punyakala and at Kurukshetra etc., holy places and the person who is ineligible to give dana or to receive dana from people, who are out casted or degraded will be affected by the diseases such as Charmaroga (skin disease), swasa, kasa, krimiroga, kandu (itching) etc . To repel this an idol of yamavahana i.e. she buffalo is to be donated depending on once ability in order to get relieved. If such practices have been done incompletely fruits will not yield both in this world and in other world as well. And also, one should chant the names of Vishnu (Vishnu Sahasra nama) and also give hiranya dana, rakta vastradana, providing meal for fifty brahmanas and bath with waters of sahasra kalasa (one thousand pots) will relieve one from the disease.

Who does not do the above donations after death getting punishments in the hell and next birth he will suffer from swasa., kasa diseases etc. To repel, he must donate sahasra pala ghrita (ghee measuring one thousand pala) will make one free from swasa.

Notes:

Dyspnoea or shortness of breath can be compared to 'Shwasa Roga' or 'Shwasa Krichrata' explained in Ayurveda. Both mean to say 'difficulty in breathing'. Generally Ayurveda use the word Swasa to describe this condition. Kasa though indicate cough but the author uses the term kasa for kapha roga.

Hikka:

Author explaining Karmavipaka of hikka mentions that

Brahmin who takes food before taking bath, homa and japa will get the hikka disease. To get rid of this sin one should perform the expiations of three chandrayana and three krichrams to get freed from the disease.

Notes:

Hiccups (hikka) are repeated spasms of diaphragm paired with a 'hic' sound produced from the vocal cords closing. Though hiccups subside normally with simple measures but it could be an indication of grave significance. Author depicted both hidhma and hikka as two separate conditions.

Prameha:

Author explaining karmavipaka of Prameha the person who undergoes sexual intercourse with woman of lower caste (chandala) develops meharoga or kshuda and pipasa roga. To repel this, he should perform chandrayana Vrata or yava madhya chandrayana or he has to perform sahasrajya sacrifice by chanting mantra (idimaapaha pravahata) etc. And also, he should perform Sacrifice with fire using ghee of one thousand pots to get relieved from the disease.

Notes:

The characteristics of Prameha is excessive urination (both in frequency & quantity) and turbidity. All prameha when not treated properly develop into madhumeha (diabetes).

Shula meha :

Author explaining Karmavipaka of Shula meha mentions that a person who does sexual intercourse with horse elephant etc., will develop sulameha. Performing santarpana etc krichras will relieve one from such disease.

Notes:

Shulameha a new disease mentioned by the author and such disease reference not available in ayurvedic texts.

Vatameha :

Author explaining Karmavipaka of Vatameha mentions that the person who indulges in sexual intercourse on days of amavasya and pournima (The day of full moon) even with his wife or with any miner girl develops the disease vatameha. Performing chandrayana prayaschitta will relieve one from such disease.

Notes :

Vatameha is also newly mentioned disease by the author. In Ayurveda texts we do not find such disease, but author might be referring to vataja prameha a disease which is incurable.

Madhumeha:

Explaining Karmavipaka of Madhumeha author mentions that

Coitus with mother causes madhumeha, and with sister causes ikshumeha. These people get relieved from these diseaes when they perform sadabda (six years), pancabdha (five years), Trayabdha (three years) Krichras .

Notes: *Just as diabetes, in Ayurveda a condition in which a person passes honey like (sweet) urine is described called Madhumeha (Hyperglycemia) .It is one among 20 types of Prameha (urological disorder) described in various Ayurvedic classics.*

Mutrakrichra: Author explaining Karmavipaka of Mutrakrichra mentions that sexual indulgence with wife of guru, or with animals makes one to get mutrakrichra. To get relieved from this disease, one has to donate three platesful of tila to get atma shuddhi.

The person who eats the food given by sudra or a person who is lazy (karmahita) will suffer from shula and ajeerna.

Notes:

Mutrakriccha is one of the diseases found in about all Ayurvedic Classics where a patient experiences painful and discomfort micturition. Mutrakriccha is of eight types having different signs and symptoms.

Asmari:

Author explaining asmari karmavipaka mentions that para stri gamana (woman other than his wife) will get apasmara (epilepsy) and asmari (calculus) . One has to do swarna dana for subsiding all types of dosa, dana are considered as best procedure.

Notes: *Asmari (Renal stones) means the presence of stone/calculus in the urinary system. Apasmara is epilepsy a condition where the person suffers from seizures (fits) .*

Ajirna sula:

शूद्रस्यैव तु भुक्तान्नमव्रतस्य द्विजस्य च । शूलव्याधिर्भवेन्नित्यं अजीर्णेनातिपीडितः ॥१॥

Person will get sula and ajirna because of taking food in the house of sudra or a brahmana who does not follow the customs.

Pleeha shula:

Author explaining karmavipaka of pleeha shula mentions that the person who poisons a person though loyal to him will develop pleeha shula .

Karmavipaka of Jathara Shula

श्रुताध्ययनसंपन्नं याचितारमकिंचनम् ॥ २

ब्राह्मणं दान्तमाहूय दानार्थं न ददाति यः । स भवेज्जठरशूली तथाध्मानी च कर्हिचित् ॥३॥ कृच्छ्रा तिकृच्छ्र चांद्राणि स कुर्याद्रोगमुक्तये ।

The person who do not donate to poor scholars of Vedas will suffer from Jathara Sula and also adhmana in their rebirth. To repel, he has to perform krichram, atikrichram, chandrayana prayaschitta (penance) .

Aruchi:

Author explaining Karmavipaka of Aruchi mentions that the person though rich but donates without respect and gives tamasa dana then he will suffer from aruchi and shula. To repel this, the patient should perform chandrayana, atikrichram, prajapatya krichram, homa etc depending on the disease and severity.

Sirah sula: Author explaining karmavipaka of Shula that the person who killed Brahmin or cow etc., in previous birth will get headache (sirah shula), earache and shula (abdominal pain).

To repel the above sin one should perform ghrita vrata for 1 year or 2 year or 3 years. Afterwards he should donate gohiranyadi (cow, deer etc) and swarna to Brahmin.

Katishula:

Author explaining Karmavipaka of Katishula mentions that the one who indulges in maithuna (coitus) with cow suffer from katishula (backache). To get rid of this one should perform kathina chandrayana and perform soura mantrajapa (muttering the names of sun god).

Notes:

Katishula is low backache, it develops due to shosha (degeneration), sthamba (stiffness), and shula (pain) of kati region and is considered as predominant vata vyadhi (disease).

Karnashula:

Author explaining Karmavipaka of Karnashula mentions that the one who hears about words of parents when they are in intimacy will have karnashula or deafness or will have annoying sound in the skull.

A Brahmin should be donated gold weighing 20 varaha, and then he should chant Vishnuprakasa mantra to get red of karnashula.

Hastashula :

Author explaining Karmavipaka of Hastashula that an atheist Brahmin in previous birth who do not perform sandhya vandana etc daily activities will get hastashula (pain in the hand). To repel this, he should donate gold weighing 12 varaha (called pagoda), and provide meal to Brahmins depending on ones capacity and chant souramantra.

Nayana shula: Explaining Karmavipaka of Nayana Shula author mentions that the person who looks to other woman when naked or the one who looks to sun both at dawn and sunset will develop pain in the eye and also develops weakness of sight.

The person who suffers from nayanashula should chant "VARAM DEHI" mantra eighty thousand times; later abhisheka is to be performed chanting "Vayassuparna" mantra.

Notes :

Description about Nayanashula and hastashula are not vailable in any Ayurveda texts. Author vallbhendra alone mentions about this. Author mentioning karmavipaka of sula and krisatva in general mentions that in order to subside this sula one has to perform annadana (donating food) and performing rudrajapa.

Gulmaroga:

Karmavipaka of gulmaroga afflicts the person who feels hatred towards guru will be afflicted by gulma. To get rid of this he should perform payovrata for one month.

Notes:

Gulma is defined as a granthi (lump) between hridaya (cardiac region) and basti (pelvic region). Vitiated vata is an invariable causative factor for all types of gulma.

The prime pathological event in gulma is the obstruction to the course of vata, which can be due to causes like inflammation, stricture, tumor etc.

Hridroga:

Author explaining Karmavipaka of hridroga mentions that the person who consumes such food (boiled rice) seen by a woman who is in menstrual period will suffer from Hridroga.

To overcome this the person should eat yava (hordeum vulgare) boiled in gomutra (cow's urine) for seven days. And also perform bheeshma panchaka and undergo fasting.

Notes:

A careful observation and a thoughtful study however reveal that in Ayurveda literature that at least two organs share almost equal claims to put themselves synonymous with the term Hridaya. At one end of the scale is the belief that Hridaya is Brain (shiro hridaya) and the other is uro hridaya (heart) ..

Udararoga:

Mentioning Karmavipaka of Udara roga that a person who gives undue importance to any one of the three gods i.e Brahma, Vishnu, Rudra will suffer from Udara.

As a penance he must perform Krichra, atikrichra, chandrayana etc expiation and also should do sahasra ghatabhisheka to god shiva to get relieved from the disease.

Notes:

Udara roga denotes generalized distension or enlargement of abdomen of any etiology. Udara roga in Ayurveda is not only limited to ascitis, accumulation of fluid in the peritoneal cavity but also includes gaseous distension, hepato-spleenomegaly of varied etiology, intestinal obstruction and intestinal perforation.

Jalodara :

राज्ञा वा तु नियुक्तेन नियुक्तो धर्मनिश्चये । पुरोहितः प्रविकस्सचिवान्यथा चरेत् ।। ३ ।। जलोदरत्वं प्राप्नोति तस्य वक्ष्यामि निष्कृतिम् ।

The persons who are supposed to uphold justice such as king, purohit, and also those who are appointed by the king or judge or minister of the royal court are not doing their jobs responsibly will suffer from Jalodara.

To repel one has to perform payovrata (drinking only milk) for three months and also perform sahasra ghatabhisheka to god Eshwara and also should provide meal to hundred brahmana to get relieved from jalodara.

Notes: *Ascites, also known as Jalodara in Ayurveda is a gastro-enterological condition of the abdomen that mainly refers to the accumulation of toxic fluid in the peritoneal cavity which chiefly leads to abdominal distension or swelling.*

Pleehodara:

Author explaining Karmavipaka of pleehodara mentions that the person who undertakes the task of teaching by taking remuneration, and the one who abuses virgin will suffer from pleehodara (splenic enlargement) . To repel this the afflicted should chant sree sookta for thirty thousand times, and to perform homa based on ruk .

Notes:

Splenomegaly or enlargement of spleen is known as 'Plihodar'. In Ayurvedic perspective liver and spleen are two organ that represents the birthplace or starting point for Rakta dhatu or blood.

Amavata:

Author explaining Karmavipaka of amavata mentions that the person who stops intentionally the fire of Havana (homagni) by pouring water will be afflicted by Amavata.

To repel this, one should chant gayatri mantra for ten thousand times .

Notes:

Ama is a maldigested product, which is not homogeneous for the body.

Amavata is a disease in which vitiation of Vata Dosha and accumulation of Ama take place in joints causing pain and inflammation in joints.This disease simulates rheumatoid arthritis (RA) in modern parlance.

Agnimandya:

Author explaining Karmavipaka of agnimandya roga mentions that

The person though possessing money but do not undertake holy or auspicious activities such as worshiping Vaisvanara etc ., gods and also do not perform homa such persons will get agnimandya roga.

To overcome the disorder one has to perform Prajapathya Krichra Traya, and also providing meal to hundred brahmanas.

But according to Parasara, Agnimandya roga will affect the persons to those who eat beef (gomamsa) . To relieve from this one should perform kathina praja patyavrata, and chant "agni gayatri " mantra & sreesukta.

At one place author gives summary of Karma Vipaka and writes that who unnecessarily poisons a person will get agnimandya disease and will take rebirth as dead. Hence he should perform ashtotthara Satahoma (One hundred and eight homa) following mate rudra sukta. Afterwards he should chant tamagnivarnam suktam one thousand times and provide meal to hundred brahmanas.

Notes:

Agnimāndya is a condition in which food is not properly digested due to the diminished power of Jaṭharāgni (digestive juices) .

Arsas: One who takes remuneration for teaching or gives remuneration to do the job of teaching or taking remuneration for conduction of homa or Japa develops arsoroga. To repel this one has to donate cow with horns covered with ½ pala of gold, and hooves made up of silver. It also should be adorned with clothes and flowers. and worshipped with sodashopachara. To please navagraha, navadhanya are kept and navagraha are worshipped chanting following mantra "Idam Vishnu hu, Prata dvishnu hu Vishnormukam either 1008 times or 108 times and also homa performed to please Vishnu. After completion of homa and poornahuti, the patient should take bath to get himself clean thus purified should give a Brahmin who is scholar of vedas and affluent in knowledge and who is peaceful must be adorned with ornaments, clothes and also with an umbrella and worship with perfumes and flowers. He should chant "govindam those manasadhyayan" mantra keeping faith in Vishnu, later he should donate gold, cow and navadhanya to get himself relieved from the disease Arsas.

Notes:

Arsha (piles) is a condition in which a fleshy mass of variable size, shape and colour appears (due to varicosity of veins) in the anus. This disease is similar to Hemorrhoides. These are swollen veins inside of the rectum or outside of anus can cause pain, anal itching and rectal bleeding.

Trishna:

Author explaining Karmavipaka of trishna mentions that the person who do not even provide water to a Brahmin, cow, or to those who are thirsty will get Trishna and Murcha diseases.

To repel this one should donate water, milk added with sugar and ghrta to brahmins with devotion will relieve one from Trishna and murcha.

Notes:

Trishna and pipasa are two commonly used words denoting desire for water, the difference between the two is, trishna is pathological and pipasa is physiological. Generally, desire for water is physiological process to maintain fluid balance but if dosha are vitiated then they can lead to excessive thirst and can produce trishna, which requires treatment.

Daha:

Author explaining Karmavipaka of daha mentions that the person who spits in the sacred fire place will get caught hold by Kapila graham and immediately will have complications like rising of fever, colicky pain, burning sensation all over the body, develops yellowish discoloration of the eyes . To repel this, he should give in sacrifies of the following such as flour, pelalu (Fried paddy), oil cake, blood gingelly seeds, aswapasha and flowers at the four road junction and chant as follows– "gruhneeshwacha balinchemam"

Notes: *The term daha generally refers to thirst but in Ayurveda it refers to aggravation of pittadosha understood as burning sensation, it is mentioned under nanatmaja pitta vikara. When pitta gets aggravated it leads to padadaha madatyaya, daha etc clinical conditions which requires to be treated with pitta hara treatement.*

Unmada:

Author explaining karmavipaka of unmada mentions that the one who intoxicates other and making them mohita (intoxicated), then he will be afflicted with unmada . To get relieved he should perform chandrayana krichra prayaschitta, saraswathi nama Japa and also he should provide meal to brahmana.

Notes:

Unmada is the major type of mental disorder considered as ubhayashraya or ubhayadhisthita vikara in ayurveda. It is the most descriptively dealt with manovikara (mental disorders) and defined as the unsettled state of manas, buddhi, sanjnajnana, smriti, bhakti, sheela, chesta and achara in Charakasamhita .

Apasmara:

ब्राह्मणश्वासारोधेन ह्यपस्मारी भवेन्नरः । वक्ष्ये तस्य प्रतीकारं दानहोक्रियाविधिम् ॥२॥ गुरौ स्वामिर्निंवास्तेयं प्रतिकूलं समाचरेत् । सोपस्मारी भवेत्तत्र कुर्याच्चांद्रायणं नरः ॥१॥

शनि भूसुतदिननाधा निधनस्था यस्य जन्मकाले स्युः । नानाव्याधिवदादैः पीडा चापस्मारसंभवां तस्य ॥ ३ ॥ अष्टमस्थानस्थित शनिमंगलसूर्यजनितापस्मारशान्तये ।

ग्रहप्रीतये पूर्वोक्तमेव सकलं जपादिकं कुर्यात् । । ४ । ।

Author explaining of Karmavipaka of Apasmara mentions that the person who steeling items of guru and is also insubordinate to his guru (master) will suffer from Apasmara. To get relieved from it chandryana prayaschitta is to be done. The person who upholds or obstructs the breathing of brahmana gets Apasmara disease. Dana and homa are to be undertaken to get relieved from the disease apasmara.

Notes : *Chandrayana, a vrata regulated by the Moon, in which the food diminishes every day by one mouthful during the dark fortnight, and similarly increases during the light fortnight.*

loss of smriti and loss of consciousness has been described as the cardinal feature of the disease Apasmara. It is similar to disease epilepsy on modern parlance.

Kusthuroga :

Author explaining Karmavipaka of kusthuroga mentions that the person who speaks harsh and also useless without any reason will get the disease Kushtu (skin disease) . To avert this he has to perform three chandrayana Krichra and also donate medicines to poor brahmins and to provide meal to brahmana depending on ones capability.

The person who indulges in sex with wife of guru or sex with animals gets the disease kustu roga. To avert this he has to perform three chandrayana.

Notes:

The term kustha generally refers to disease leprosy but in Ayurveda it indicates all types of skin diseases, which includes leprosy also. Kushtha Chikitsa is a compendium of various skin diseases, divided into two groups i.e. major (maha kushtha) and minor (kshudra kushtha) . Seven types of major and eleven types of minor skin disorders or dermatosis are described here as guidelines to understand diagnosis and treatment principles of various skin disorders.

Galaganda:

Author explaining Karmavipaka of galaganda mentions that the person who steals galagandee gana dravya will get galagandaroga. To avert this one should prepare a necklace with rubies, diamond, vaidhurya, neela, marakata. If some of them are lacking he should procure the maximum number of available things kept in order using silver thread and should keep them in a copper utensil filled with gingelly seeds. Navagraha are to be worshipped keeping this utensil infront of idols. Later this utensil is donated to a scholarly Brahmin.

Guru (the master) who deceivingly teaches the student, or the student deceivingly learns the subject from guru will get the disease galaganda. Apart from this, those who eat which is inedible or intoxicants will also get afflicted by the disease. To repel this, the afflicted must undertake three kricha, chandrayana, and chanting purusha sukta for one thousand eight times and perform soura mantra, and also he should provide meals to Brahmin to get relieved from the disease.

Notes:

The disease Galaganda is explained by Charaka, Susruta and Vagbhata as a swelling around the neck region. Taking into consideration the site, size and features as well this disease entity has been compared to hypothyroidism, which involves certain features of swelling, heaviness etc.

Gandamala is a pathological condition, which presents as swelling in the neck. While Galaganda is a single swelling occurring on the side of the neck, gandamala is a series of similar swellings in the neck, which looks like a garland of swellings.

Sleepada: Author explaining Karmavipaka of Sleepada mentions that the person who indulges sex with woman of one's own gotra will be afflicted with sleepada, and the woman who undergoes sex with her own gotra will get bleeding per vagina. To avert this one should perform chandrayana praysachitta and payovrata for one month.

They should donate an idol having three feet (tripada) holding dhanus, knife and falling down posture is to be donated.

Notes:

Filariasis was well known to ancient Indians by the name Shlipada. It is described that the word Shlipada must be understood as an increase in the size of the foot. The word 'Shlipada' is derived from "shilavat padam shlipadam", where the limb/foot becomes hard like stone.

Vrana roga:

Author explaining Karmavipaka of Vrana Roga mentions that the person who indulges sex with woman of upper caste will take birth having siro vrana. To get purified one has to perform prajapathya vrata.

At the auspicious hour of performing sandhya vandana etc if any person looks at hen or donkey will suffer from nasika Vrana (nasal Ulcer) and watering of eyes. To repel, he should follow udyannadye with sahasra charu ahuti and srisukta japa. Then by following sivasankalpa, abhimantrita durva and akshata should be tied in his hair.

Notes: *Acharya Sushruta has explained that vrana (wounds/ulcers) is a condition of destruction of tissues or the process or event by which destruction of the tissues occur and after healing it leaves a scar on that area or part and it remains the same whole life.*

Nadivrana:

Author explaining Karmavipaka of Nadivrana mentions that the person who inflicts injury to Vrana of other person with blows, or the one who lies will get birth afflicted by pleeha, asteela and naadivrana. To repel this he has to perform chandrayana, atikrichram, pratichandrayana vrata, atiroudra, sukta by giving 108 ahuti, kushmanda homa etc.,, thereafter ten sahasra japa of varuna has to be performed.

Notes: *Nadi Vrana is a name given to describe Sinus occuring in anal region or any other region. Fistula in ano can also be included under Nadi Vrana (though Bhagandara is a name given for Ayurvedic version of anal fistula).*

Pleeha indicates increase of size of spleen. The anatomical position of the prostate gland is described in Ayurvedic classic Yogaratnakara as – Below umbilicus (naabhi), it is a hard gland which is little bit bulged and changes its place like "ashteela" (a small stone used to sharpen swords). This gland, when affected by vitiated Vata, causes a disease called "Vathaashteela" this condition are comparable to Benign prostate hypertrophy.

Bhagandara :

Author explaining karmavipaka of Bhagandhara (fistula in ano) mentions that the person who performs coitus with a lady belongs to his own gotra will get bhagandhara. In order to subside this bhagandhara that person should donate idol of mesa (goat) made with gold and silver while chanting the mantra.

Upadamsa:

Author explaining Karmavipaka of Upadamsa (sexually transmitted disease) mentions that indulging sex with chandala (out caste) brings in Sweta kustu. To repel this kalasa (pot) has to be palced west to the fire place, and an idol of kubera wrapped in with black cloth and adorned with flowers and garlands then daily it is worshipped with shodashopachara, Parayana of adharvana Veda is to be done in front of it every day. This idol has to be donated while chanting "Vidheena Madhipo devatyadi mantra" will relieve one from heena kusta and linganasa.

Mukha roga (diseases of the face and oral cavity) :

Person who gives wrong evidence gets mukharoga and raktapitta roga. To avert ati kathina chandrayana vrata, thereafter kushmanda homa and gayatri japa has to be performed. Then gold and grains are to be donated.

Karna roga (ear disease) :

The person who deliberately hears abusing parents, guru devata and brahmana such people will suffer from bleeding and also discharge of pus from ear. To avert this four krichravrata has to be performed. After this, gold red cloth should be donated to brahmin. Soura mantra Japa and homa are to be performed.

Kasa:

The one who steals the money of poor by deceiving them will get the disease kasa. To repel this, measures of penance such as santarpana, krichra are to be performed.

II. The one who steals tin will develop Kapharoga. To repel this one should fast for one day and on the next day he should donate 400 tulas of tagara (tin).

III. The person who abandons once daily rituals develops Kapharoga and also gets insulted by the foes. To get rid of this the afflicted person should eat yavakaanna, chant Vishnu sahasranama and perform homa avatudal (Naama mantrena kurveeta charvajyam cha havirbhavet). It appears author uses kapharoga as a synonym for kasa.

Notes :

Author used the term kapharoga to indicate respiratory diseases.

Yavakanna is the rice prepared from yava.

Prāyaścitta is the Sanskrit word which means "atonement, penance, expiation". In Hinduism, it is a dharma-related term and refers to voluntarily accepting one's errors and misdeeds, confession, repentance, means of penance and expiation to undo or reduce the karmic consequences. In this process preparing an idol of god and worshipping it, giving donations to Brahmins, performing homa and chanting soura mantra, gayatrimantra etc., are done as part of ritual. The concept of vratas date back to the Ṛgveda, and it refers to self-imposed restrictions on food and behavior, sometimes with a vow.

JYOTISSASTRABHIPRAYAM (ASTROLOGICAL CONSIDERATIONS) AS A CAUSATION OF DISEASE.

Astrological consideration as the cause for disease is a new contribution by the author. They are as follows.

At birth time if the place of surya is in Karkataka rasi (zodiac sign of cancer) and afflicted by the vision of sani (Saturn) gets vata disease. Then his nature will be like a thief, and posses unstable mind and he will be backbiting by nature.

If a person's birth time Ketu's presence is in sani madhyama, then he will be affected by vata pitta roga. He will have strife with lower caste and will tend to proceed to go other countries.

The person if takes birth at the time when angaraka (mars) is present in chandrakshetra (candra kshetra) will be afflicted by the diseases Raktapitta (bleeding disease) and Durnamaroga. In another verse author writes that the afflicted person will have complications with fire and air. In order to pacify, the afflicted should chant angaraka mantra and lit sacrificial fire with Chandra fuel sticks and tila (gingily seeds) . Later the patient should donate Vrishabha having blood colour in order to get cured of the diseases.

To pacify the bad effects of the astronomical disorder he also prescribes a kashaya prepared from bilva, chandana, bala sanapushpa, inguleeka, Vakula phalaniseha for internal use, and the patient is also advised to take bath with this kashaya.

At the time of birth, presence of Krura graham is in their natural dwelling place or if the presence of krura graham in the gurusthana such person will be affected by mandagni (low digestive fire), such person will get defeated in the war, and will have prejudiced mind, tendency for sinful acts arise. To repel this one should resort to japa, homa and snana etc activities.

Notes:

The Krura Grahas in a horoscope are the harbinger of all troubles in life. The chief among them is Shani. The other Krura grahas are Mangal, Rahu and Ketu.

At the time of birth if Chandra and sukra are present in the 6th house or having their vision on them. Then such person gets afflicted with chardhi or Trishna. Budha being in 6th place and if sees depleting Chandra, in him either of the disease chardhi or Trishna (vomiting and thirst respectively) develop.

At whose birth time surya happens to be in karkataka rasi, and under the influence of vitiated glimpse of Budha, such person develops blindness, kapharoga and vataroga. Such person will have the attitude of stealing and also develops fickle mindedness.

At whose birth time, sani is in the seventh place and is associated with Rahu then such person will get the disease mutra krichra (difficulty in urination).

At whose janma laghna Chandra possess papagraha Madhya sthithi and sani sthithi in seventh house, then such person will get swasa, Kshaya, vidradhi (abcess), gulma (hard mass like tumor) and pleeha (enlargement of spleen diseases).

At the time of birth if mangalagraha placed in the dasama sthana (tenth house) and if the person is looked by sani (Saturn) then such person will get vatarakta (gout).

To pacify vitiated rakta dosha one should satisfy Angaraka by doing Japa and homa. At the time of whose Janma Laghna (In a birth chart, the Lagna refers to the ascending sign at the time of birth of an individual at a particular place. Lagna literally means connection, referring to the beginning of an individual's life.) If brihaspati resides in the astamasthana (eight house) then such person suffers from Amavata. To repel this japa, dana, puja and homa are to be performed.

नीचस्थितस्यदूंनाशबंधपीडाःभानोर्भवतिकुष्ठस्यदशायांज्वरशिशरोरोगः ॥ १३ ॥

च श्रदर्शनंश्चित्रम् ।क्षीर्णेंदुदशायामप्येवं । सुहृद्बंधुसमायोगो । सुहृद्बंधुसमायोगो भूनिमित्तं कलिर्भवेत् ॥ १४ ।देहपीडा ज्वरो व्याधिशिशखिमध्यगते बुधे । शनेरंतर्गतेऽप्येवं ज्योतिशशास्त्रविनिश्चयः ॥ १५ ॥तद्वैकृतनिरासाय जपहोममा दिकं चरेत् ।

If surya (sun) stays in neecha kshetra in dasamadhyama then the person will get fever, head related problems, losing of eyes, bandhana, pida (pain), switra (lukoderma) and other skin diseases (kusta). If Chandra is in ksina desa also, this disease occur.

A person having ketu dasa madhyama Budhantaradasa he meet with friends and relatives. Land related problems will occur and also suffers from body pains and jwara. In case of sani antardasa also similar situation occurs. To avoid these entire one has to perform japa and homa.

At the time of birth if sani Angaraka Surya reside in eigth place, then any of the disease or the apasmara will occur. To relieve this, measures such as to pleasing graha homa Japa are to be undertaken.

ASHTA STHANA PARIKSHA

Author Vallabhacharya begins his book Vaidya cintamani with the chapter "Ashtasthana Pariksha" (eight fold method of clinical examination) shows the importance he has given for clinical diagnosis.

According to Ayurveda, Rogi pariksa or the examination of a patient consists of three steps: Darsana (examination by inspection), Sparsana (examination by touch) and Prasna (examination by interrogation).

A sharp observation of the patient's gait, physique and appearance conveys a lot of information about his general condition. This is called "darsana pariksa" or observation.

"Sparsana pariksa" is the examination by touch (sparsa). The physician can evaluate several factors through the medium of touch. He can assess the temperature of the body, feel the margins of swellings in skin, read and note the characteristics of pulse, or check for organ enlargements.

For an overall picture of the illness, a detailed interrogation (prasna pariksa) of the patient and his family member or relative is necessary. Gathering information by putting specific questions about symptoms, lifestyle, diet and medical history and systematically observes other features that may provide clues to the cause and duration of the illness.

Darsana, sparsana and prasna together comprise "Trividha Pariksa" - the threefold method of clinical examination. An elaborative version of the above is the "Astavidha Pariksa" or the eightfold method of patient examination by the author Vallabhacharya. Astasthana pariksa includes the following eight factors: Nadi (pulse), Mala (frequency, color, consistency of bowel movements), Mutra (urine - color, frequency, burning sensations), Jihva (tongue), Sabda (voice and speech of the patient), Sparsa (touch, skin and tactile sense), Drik (eyes and vision), and Akriti (general body build, eg: lean, obese, muscular, etc.) .

Though "Ashtasthana Pariksha" of Vaidya cintamani appears similar to that mentioned in treatises like Yogaratnakara and Sarangadhara (most renowned treaties of Ayurveda belong to 17th century A.D.) But on close scrutiny it reveals that asthasthana pareeksha of vaidya chintamani differs with them in many aspects.

Nadi:

Notes :

Pulse implies Nadi in Sanskrit. The earliest evidence about Nadi Pariksha are found mainly in texts namely Bhela Samhita and in Harita Samhita. In modern medicine physician gets important information like rate, rhythm, pressure, force by examining pulse. But in Ayurveda the importance of Nadi Parkisha is to understand pathogenesis, diagnosing of diseases and also to assess prognosis of the disease.

In Asthavidh Prakisha, Nadi Pariksha is most important since it assess Prakruti, Vikruti, Doshic disorder and also prognosis of disease. Nadi pariksha (examination of the pulse) is to be examined in hand and leg of the patient. The pulse below the thumb and the pulse at the root of the leg is examined. Vata, Pitta, & Kapha circulate in whole body producing well or ill consequences in entire body according to their state of increase or decrease. Their normal state is Prakruti and their abnormal state is Vikruti. All three Dosha move in body through Rasa and Rakta Dhatu. We can feel qualities of Vata best under index finger, Pitta under middle and Kapha under ring finger.

1) Measuring size of Nadi :

आदौ समस्तरोगेषु हाष्टस्थानं परीक्षयेत् । नाड़ी स्पर्शश्च रूपञ्च शब्दञ्च नेत्रे पुरीषकं ॥ ११ ॥ मूत्रवगच जिह्वांच होतान्यश्येद्विषग्वरः । अंगुष्ठमूलमाश्रित्य ह्यंगुलीत्रयमात्रिका ॥ १२ ॥ यवबीजप्रमाणेन नाडीसर्वांगसंगता।

Nadi present below angusta (thumb) mula in the measurement of three angula equal to the size of yava bija will provide the status of the total body.

2) Naadi (pulse) :

करमूले पादमूले नाडी वहति दृश्यताम् ॥ १३ ॥

नारीणां वामभागे च पुंसां दक्षिणभागके । वातपित्तयस्यापि श्लेष्मणश्च गतिस्तथा ।। १४ ।। यथानाडी तथाचर्या विज्ञेया वैद्यपारगैः ।

Physician should examine the pulse below the thumb and at the root of the leg. On the left side for female and right side for male pulse is to be examined.

वातनाडीवक्रगतिर्भेकलावुकसर्पवत् ॥ १५ ॥

चपला पित्तनाडी च गच्छेन्मंडूकबर्हिवत् ।। १६ ॥

लस्य डोलिकाभा च जलूका या गतिर्भवेत् ।

(pittaja nadi)

पारावातगतिश्चापि कपोतगति सन्निभा । कफात् स्थिरगतिर्नाडी कुक्कुटस्य गतिर्यथा ॥ १७।

मरालस्येव चटकाटिट्टिभ्योश्च गतिर्यथा । (kaphaja nadi)

क्षणे विषधरस्येव क्षणे मंडूकबर्हिवत् ॥ १८ ॥

वातपित्तगतिं प्राहुर्विज्ञेय च भिषग्वरैः । (vatapitta nadi)

क्षणे लावुकवद्गच्छेन्मरालगमना क्षणे ॥ १९॥

वातश्लेष्मयुता नाडी विज्ञेया च भिषग्वरैः । (vata sleshma nadi)

क्षणे कुक्कुटवद्गच्छेत्क्षणे गच्छेन्मयूरवत् ॥ २० ॥

पित्तश्लेष्मगतिज्ञेयां वैद्यविद्याविशारदैः ॥ (pitta sleshma nadi)

3) Assessing dosha movement by naadi: Author of the view that both Vata pitta naadi move below the first finger and selshma nadi under the middle finger. The pulse reading should be done according to dosha order. The physician also should collect the information about patient dinacharya (Dinacharya in Ayurveda refers to the daily activities people need to perform to stay healthy).

4) The characteristics of dosha gati lakshanas in Vaidya chintamani differ with other ayurvedic texts. For instance in Vataja Naadi We find a new set of symptoms than those mentioned in sarangadhara Samhita and Bhavaprakasha. He explained that Vata nadi will have Vakra gati and the movement will be similar to bheka (frog), lavaka bird (leg movements), Sarpa (snake), Jalaga (leach). Another striking description by vallbhendra that in vata pradhana nadi will be like "Balasya dolabhavana" (Swing of baby).

While describing pitta nadi we find new contributions such as the naadi of pitta will be chanchala (unstable), and moves like mayura (peacock), and kapota (pigeon). He skips kaka (crow) and manduka (frog) gati mentioned in Yogaratnakara and Sarangadhara.

While describing kapha naadi Vallabhacharya gives us extra description like kapota (pigeon), maral (swan) and will have movement like tittibha. The lakshanas mentioned for sleshma described in other texts are found for pitta naadi in vaidya chintamani.

In Sarangadhara and yogarathnakara there is mere indication of dwandwaja lakshnas (mixed characteristics of 2 doshas.) But we find elaborative description of dwandwaja dosa naadi lakshanas in vaidya chintamani. It is striking to note that selshma pitta naadi will be like snake in the beginning but in short time attains movement as peacock. And describing Vata pitta naadi that it will be sluggish and will have the movement like snake to start with but will have the movement of peacock or frog in short period. Describing vatasleshma nadi author states that the movement will be like lavaka bird to begin with but later attains movement of maral (swan) . This kind of accurate description of dwandwaja nadi reveals his efforts to standardise dosagati movements by naadi pariksha clinically .

Another striking contribution of indrakanthi vallabhacharya is mentioning about the characteristics of nadi diseasewise.

सुप्तकाको यथा गच्छेत्तथा स्त्रीसंपगमे स गति । हंसवन्मंदगा नाडी विज्ञेया मलबंधके ॥ २२ ॥ (ajirna nadi lakshana)

काष्ठभारस्य मध्ये तु मूषिकागमनं यथा । कुटिलं शिथिलं मंदं सूक्ष्मं च चपलं तथा ॥ २३ । । सन्निपाताद्रतिं नाड्या विजानीयाद्विषम्वरः । Sannipata lakshana)

भुक्ते च स्नानमात्रे च निद्रिते चाप्युपोषिते ॥ २४॥ व्यायामक्लान्तदेहे च भूताविष्टे सरोदने । सुंदरीभिश्च संयुक्ते मद्यपाने मतिभ्रमे ॥ २५ ॥

पवनायामसाधने । शशकुक्कुटमंडूकसर्पमांसादिभक्षणे ॥ २६ ॥

गांधारीभक्षणे चैव अपस्मारक्लांतदेहे नाडी सम्यङ् न बुध्यते ।
नाडीगतिमविज्ञाय चिकित्सां तनु ते तु यः ॥ २७॥ स रोगी नरकं याति विजानानो भिषग्वरः । (samsayana nadi akshna).

The following are the characteristics of nadi in the following disease.

Characteristics of nadi	Clinical Condition
The movement of elephant	Ajeerna
Crow which is not having sleep	When food which not got digested.
Movement similar to rat moving in between large collection of sticks have pulse sometimes similar to the movement of curved and within a short period pulse changes to sithila (weak), and sometimes attains mandagati (slow movement) and sometime attains sukshma (feeble).	Sannipata nadi
Slow movement of Swan	Constipation.

Notes:

According to Ayurveda tridosha (vata, pittaand kapha are considered as three fundamental biological energies. These doshas are accountable for the homeostasis and the health of living beings. When these energy forces are in state of equilibrium the living beings are in normal health status and when they are deviate produce diseases. When these tridoshas are abnormal produce some specific characteristics. These are expressed in the form of symptoms and signs and also as abnormalities of pulse.To recognize them nadi pariksha is essential.

Sannipatika means 'conglomeration of vitiated tridosa (vata, pitta and kapha)' is of manifested disease.

The description of the movement as crow not having sleep and the movement of elephant are difficult for analysis and comprehension.

The characteristic of sannipata nadi is not only amazing but also its meticulous descriptions by the author is rewarding. According to him sannipata nadi will be like rodent moving in between the logs of wood and will have movement such as Vakra (crooked or curved), kutilam, sithilam, mandam, sukshmam and chapalam (crooked, collapsed, sluggish, minute and unstable respectively).

Samsayana Nadi: Author stating about samsaya nadi (nadi not cearly understood) that in some conditions nadi will not be felt properly hence the correct state of the clinical condition can not be identified. According to author in the following conditions such as who has taken meal, after bath, who has just woken up, fasting, who walked long distances, tired, caught by devils, undergone sexual intercourse, who drank alcohol, who has taken bhang, while on yoga exercises, who has eaten meat, epilepsy, in them the pulse will not run properly.

Hence reading pulse in such conditions only lead to improper diagnosis. Basing on this false state of naadi if one resorts to treatment will only accrue the sin of the patient because of which he got the disease.

Sparsa (Palaption) :

अथ स्पर्शमिमं वक्ष्ये किंचिदुष्णं प्रभंजने ॥ २८ ॥

अत्युष्णं पित्तरोगे तु ह्यथवा चातिशीतलम् । किंचिच्छीतं श्लेष्मरोगे द्वंद्वजे च
यथायथम् ॥ २९ ॥

Notes: *Palpation is the process of feeling an object in or on the body to determine its size, shape, firmness, or location, tenderness and temperature etc. by using hands.*

In the condition of vata pradhana sparsa, it will be little usna (hot), Where as in the pitta pradhana roga it will be more usna (very hot), in the case of kapha roga, sparsa will be little sitala (cold). In case of dwandwaja roga sparsa will be according to two dosa.

Rupa (general appearance) :

ततःस्वरूपं पश्येद्वै श्यामाभं च प्रभंजने । हरिद्रं रक्तवर्णं वा गात्रं पित्ते
विनिर्दिशेत् ॥ ३० ॥

बंधके ॥२२॥ (rupa lakshana)

Notes: *Inspection (general appearance) should begin with the patient's general appearance, state of nutrition, symmetry, and posture. Wasting and hallmarks of poor nutrition other signs of disease which indicate disease; poor grooming or slack posture may suggest depression or low self-esteem.*

In yogaratnakara and Bhavaprakasa we get different term for this as "Akriti" for rupa. Rupa though appear similar to Akriti it (rupa) it also indicates about the symptoms of the disease. In vata it is syama varna (black colour), in pitta pradhana it is haridra varna (turmeric colour) or rakta varna (red colour). In the condition of kapha pradhana patient will appear pandu varna (white colour) and misrita (mixed) in dwandwaja pradhana dosa .In sannipatika pradhana the patient body will appear in *vivarna (discoloration)*.

Sabda (sound/speech):

शारदैःततः शब्दगुणं वक्ष्ये समशब्दः समीरणे। हर्षी चोल्बणवाक्पैत्ते
श्लेष्मरोगे च हीनवान्।। ३२।।

Notes:

In present days auscultation (heard by stethoscope) is performed for the purposes of examining normal and abnormal sounds of the circulatory and respiratory systems (heart and breath sounds) as well as the alimentary canal. In Ayurveda it is mainly restricted to abnormalities of speech.

Though author includes sadba as part of clinical examination similar to other texts, but gives totally different characteristics of sabda for dosha when compared to brihatrayee. These are as follows:

Vatarogi	-	simple voice
Pittarogi	-	harsha and ulvana sabda (joy and high pitch)
Kapharogi (brihatrayi deep	-	manda sabda (feeble voice) and profound speech mentioned.)
Dwandwaja	-	Mixed Speech

Netra (examination of the eye): The following are the new contributions made by the author with regard to the characteristics of netra of the atient,

Vata rogi - Shyama (black), Suna (Oedematic), Sravana (oozing)

Pitta rogi	-	Yellowish or reddish in colour
Kapha rogi	-	Matting, white in colour
Sannipata	-	yellowish and red colour
Kamila	-	Yellowish

Pureesa (examination of stool) :

पुरीषलक्षणं वक्ष्ये पवमाने च बद्धविट् ॥ ३६ ॥

अथवा श्यामला विट् स्यात्पित्ते हारिद्ररक्तम् । पिच्छिलं वा क्वचित्प्रोक्तं मलं श्लेष्मणि कफेऽनिलम् ॥

आमे वा श्लेष्मणा तुल्यं द्वंद्वजे मिश्रितं भवेत् ॥ (purisa Pariksha)

The word pureesa is being used for mala.

The following characteristic features of pureesa are his unique contributions and many of these features are contrary to other Ayurvedic texts.

Characteristic of Pureesa

Vata rogi	-	Black, Constipated
Pitta rogi	-	turmeric or red in colour
Sleshma rogi	-	white or frothy or sticky
Dwandwaja	-	mixed colour
Kamila	-	Yellowish

Note:

Vitiation of vata, pitta and kapha causes above said features in stool when they are in in abnormal conditions . Many a time author misses Sannipata category (All doshas in mixed condition) the order that is generally followed by brihatrayee (caraka, susruta and Vagbhata) most probably due to its practical difficulty in identifying sannipata condition.

Mutra (examination of urine):

वायौ च पांडुरं मूत्रं रक्तवर्णं च पैत्तिके । अथवा पीतवर्णं च कामिलाया तथैव च ॥ ३९ ॥

ततो मूत्रपरीक्षा च वक्ष्यते शास्त्रनिश्चिता ॥ ३८ ॥

श्वेतवर्णं कफे चैव द्वंदजे मिश्रितं भवेत् ॥

In this examination also we find authors own contribution with reference to urine. They are as follows:

Vata rogi: White colour of urine (pandu varna) (contrary to ayurvedic texts)

Pitta rogi   -   Red colour (instead of yellow colour)

Kamila   -   Yellow colour

Sleshma rogi   -   White and frothy

Dwandwarogi   -   Colours are mixed.

Note:

Yellowish discolouration usually found in pittarogi, and it is not mentioned here, but this feature is exclusively attributed to the disease kamala (jaundice) . The category of sannipata is missing and the features of sannipata are attributed to dwandhawa rogi. In dwandwa also he did not specify about what type of dwandhwaja (eg. Vata pitta, pitta kajha, and vata kapha) he was referring to in the text Vaidyacintamani.

Jihwa (examination of tongue) :

जिह्वा पीता स्फोटखरास्पष्टामारुतलक्षणा ॥ ४० ॥श्यावा शोणा भवेत्पित्ते
श्वेता जिह्वा, द्रवा कफे । सकंटा च शुष्का च सान्निपातिकलक्षणा ॥४१॥
मिश्रवर्णा भवेज्जिह्वा द्वंदजे परिकीर्तिता । एवं परीक्ष्य वैद्यस्तु
पश्चात्कुर्याच्चिकित्सितम् ॥४२॥

Following are the different characteristic features mentioned for Jihwa by the author, and these can be considered as his contribution. According to him when tridosha become abnormal in person the following abnormal features develop.

Vata rogi (Peeta (yellowish), Visphota yukta); Pitta rogi (Black or Red Colour); Sleshma rogi (White colour and possess moisture); SannipataKantaka, Suska (thorny, dry) and black in colour and in dwandawarogi Colours are mixed

SALIENT FEATURES OF DISEASES MENTIONED IN VAIDYACINTAMANI

Jwara

ज्वरः सप्तविधः प्रोक्तो वातात्पित्तात्कफात्तथा ॥ २० ॥

भूतो जीर्णाभिघातेभ्यो द्वंदाच्च परिकीर्तितः ॥

In Vaidya Chintamani we observe mention of different types of classification of Jwara. According to him Jwara is classified into 7 types at the first instance. They are Vata, Pitta, Kapha, Bhuta, Ajeerna, Abhighata and Dwandwaja.

Generally he misses Tridoshaja Jwara and Agantu Jwara, but adds up Bhuta Jwara and Ajeerna Jwara and dwandwaja Jwara. Dwandwaja jwara is depicted as one. The symptoms mentioned for Jwara differ with brihatrayee in toto. We find another unique classification of Jwara by the author i.e. Samanaya Jwara, Maha Jwara, Rudra Jwara and Vaisnava Jwara. No such classification is available in any other ayurvedic text.

In Vaidya chintamani author puts forward a different symptomatology for each Jwara. It is as follows. (Symptoms, which differ, are mentioned here under)

Vata Jwara: Krishna Varnam Mukham, Kandu, Timira, Shyava twak, nakha, netra and mala and pain in the head.

Pitta Jwara: Atinidrata (nidralpatvam mentioned in Madhavanidana), Rakta mutra pureeshata (yellowish discolouration mentioned in Madhavanidana)

Kapha Jwara: Pandu, panchavidha twagadisha, Hrillepa, Urdhuva Swasa

The causative factors mentioned for abhighataja Jwara are tiresomeness due to walking long distances or due to exercise, desire for taking meal, body becoming cool.

All the above symptoms are not mentioned in any Ayurvedic texts. Interestingly there is no mention of injury as the causative factor of Jwara.

Apart from usual symptoms of Vata pitta jwara, Vatasleshma, pitta sleshma, Sleshma pitta some important symptoms mentioned in the following jwaras.

Ajirṇa Jwara Lakṣaṇa

ज्वरश्च गुंभनं हिक्का मंदाग्निर्जानुनिव्यथा ।
आम्लस्वाभाविकोद्गारावजीर्णज्वरलक्षणम् ॥ ४२ ॥

Jwara (Fever), Adhmāna (Flatulance with gurgling sound), Hikka (Hiccup), Mandāgni (Dyspepsia), Janupida (Pain in the Knee joint), Amlodgāra (Acid erectation/ Belching) and Ajīrna (Dyspepsia) are the Ajīrna jwara laksana.

Abhighāta Jwara:

अध्वव्यायामतश्चैव जायते ज्वरउत्कटः । तृष्णा सर्वांगवैकल्यं
स्वेदसंतापविभ्रमम् ॥ ४३ ॥ शीतलं भोजने वांछा ह्याभिघातज्वराकृतिः

Fever increases because of continous walking and exercise, Tṛṣṇa (Thirst), Sarvanga pīda (Pain all over the body), Sweda (Sweating), Santāpa (Rise in body temparature), Bhrama (Vertigo) and intension to take cold food are the Abhighata Jwara Lakṣana.

Bhutajwara:

अपस्मारो विरूपादर्श्वर उग्रः प्रलापनम् ॥ ४४ ॥

अतीभोजने वांछा रोमहर्ष गाथनम्। हास्यं च नर्तनं तंद्रास्याद्भूतज्वरलक्षणम् ॥ ४५ ॥

Apasmāra (Epilepsy), Viripa (Ugly), Tivra jwara (Severe fever), Pralāpa (De- lirium), Intension to take more food, Romaharsa (Erection of the hair of the body followed by excitement), Singing, Loughing, Dancing, Tandra (Drowsiness) are the Bhita Jwara Laksana.

Ateeva Bhojana Vancha – (excessive desire for taking meal)

Hasyam cha nartanam (laughing and dancing) This type of Jwara though not mentioned separately but included in abhishanga Jwara in other texts.

Ahika Jwara:

अतः परं प्रवक्ष्यामि ह्याहिकज्वरलक्षणम्। शीतं सपुलकं कासतृष्णासन्तापदूयुजः ॥ ४६ ॥ शिरोरुगंगवैकल्यं कुक्षिपार्श्व सशूलकम्। अपथ्यवांछा तंद्रा च पादहन्मुखशोभकः ॥ ४७ ॥ गात्रं पांडुरवर्णं च पीतवर्णे च लोचने। नखवर्त्में च नीरक्तं ह्यतिसारश्च जाड्यकम् ॥ ४८ ॥ करपादविदाहश्च ह्याहिकज्वरलक्षणम्।

This particular Jwara is another contribution by the author. Important symptoms include white colour (paleness) of the body but yellowish discolouration of the eyes.

Desire for taking food, which are not conducive to health.

Pata hrinmulja Spbhakam (swelling, bloodlessness in nails and lids

(Nakha pakshamcha neeraktam)

Ahika Jwara Laksana:

Sita (Feeling of cold), Pulakan (Romaharsa (Erection of the hair of the body fol- lowed by excitement), Kasa (Cough), Trsna (Thirst), Santāpa (Increased Temperature), Mutra pida (Pain during micturation), Sira śūla (Headache), Angapīda (Pain in the body parts), Kuksisula (Pelvic pain), Intension to take Apathya āhara (Diet which is not indicated), Tandra (Drowsiness), Padaśotha (Inflammetion in the foot), Hrdaya Sotha (In- flammation in the Heart), Mukhaśotha (Inflammation in the mouth), Pandu Varna (Pale white colour in different parts of body), Yellow colouration of eye, Rakta hinata in Vartma (Presence of less blood in the conjuctiva of eye lid), Atisāra (Diarrhoea), Jādyata (Stiff- in foot) are the Ahika Jwara Laksana (Characters) . Hastadāha (Burning sensation in hands), Pādadāha (Burning sensation

Different names of Ahika Jwara

ऐकाहिकं द्वाहिकं च त्र्याहिकं च चतुर्थकम् ॥ ४९ ॥

पंचाहिकं चार्धपक्षं पाक्षिकं मासिकं तथा । वातपित्तश्लेष्मदोषैज्वरं विद्याद्द्विषग्वरः ॥५०

Ahika Jwara as Ekahika, dwyahika, Tryahika, Chaturdhika, panchahika, ardhapaksam, pakshikam and masika jwara. These jwaras named depending on the time it recurs. (Fever occurring at scheduled days like every 15 days (pakshikam), 30 days (masikam etc) .

Viṣama Jwara Lakṣaṇa:

क्षणे शीतं क्षणे चोष्णं क्षणेऽपि ज्वर उत्कटः । । ६५॥

क्वचिन्निद्रा न वा स्वापो द्वितीयेऽहिंज्वरः क्वचित् । ज्वरश्चातुर्थिको वापि
विषमज्वरलक्षणम् ॥ ६६ ।

Santata etc Jwara: In major Ayurvedic texts these jwaras mentioned under Vishama Jwara. In Vaidya chintamani we do get reference of vishama Jwara at one place but lacks its original definition. Apart from this, Even characteristics of these santata, satata, anyedyuka, Triteeyaka, chaturdhaka Jwara are different when compared to jwaras mentioned in brihatrayee (Caraka, Susruta, Vagbhata) . The term anyedyuka used instead for anyedyuska.

He did not mention pralepaka Jwara and vata balasaka Jwara.

Notes :

Vagbhata mentions that the fever which has the below mentioned characteristics is called as vishama jwara .

Vishama arambha – (abrupt / bizarre beginning) – fever begins abruptly, sometimes from the head and sometimes from the back and so on

Vishama kriya (bizarre activity) – sometimes there will be excessive cold associated with fever and sometimes with lot of heat

Vishama kala (uneven distribution of duration of fever) – here the time of attack of fever and duration of suffering needs to be considered. The time and days of attack of anyedhyushka, tritiyaka and chaturthaka fevers are abrupt. In these types of irregular fevers, the fever can manifest before or after the expected time and day of their appearance. Similarly the duration of fever too may be abrupt. Sometimes the fever persists for a short duration and other times for longer duration.

Dhatugata Jwara:

The fevers which are deep seated inside one or the other tissue i.e rasa, rakta, mamsa, medo, asthi, majja, sukra in a stubborn way are called as dhatugata jwaras.

Though author describes dhatugata Jwara, but the symptoms of these jwara totally differ with those mentioned in briha trayee. The term sukla is frequently used to denote sukra.

Murcha Jwara:

ज्वराणां दारुणानां च भीष्मो मूर्छा ज्वरो भवेत् । प्रवर्तते यदा शीतं तदा तंद्रा ज्वरोग्रता

ज्वरोत्पत्तिस्तथा मूर्छा सत्त्वःहानिशिरो भ्रमः । हीनस्स्वरश्चातिसारः प्रलापो बहुभाषणम् ॥ १८२ ॥ मुखे च शोषस्सर्वांगे शूलं मूत्रस्य निस्स्नुतिः । जिह्वा वदन तिक्तत्वं श्वासोत्पत्तिश्च शीतकम् ॥ १८३ ॥ नेत्रं स्रवति तोयं च करपादं च शीतलम् । रक्ताक्षिरक्तमूत्रत्वं मूर्च्छेज्वरसमुद्भवे ॥ १८४ ॥ जोगीरसः प्रयोक्तव्यो मूर्छाज्वरहरः परः । त्यक्त्वा तरुणतां नित्यं त्रिकालं ग्रंथिधान्यकम् । वरालं माक्षिकयुतं भपतिर्वीरिविक्रमः ॥ १८५ ॥

We find a unique description i.e Murcha Jwara. It states that when the patient experience coolness, then he will get tandra (drowsiness), after that the fever subsides. When fever subsides murcha completely gets vanished. This Jwara considered as dosa Jwara Sama and is analogue of death and it suffers the human beings at the end of their lives.

Notes: *Murcha a clinical condition generally refers to fainting or syncope which leads to unconsciousness for a brief period. Here this probably meant about unconsciousness generally occurs before death.*

Sita Jwara Lakṣaṇa:

शीतं कंपो भ्रमोत्यर्थं रोमहर्षो विजृंभणम् ॥ ६९ ॥

शिरःकट्यूरुपार्श्वार्तिः पिंडिकोद्वेष्टनं क्लमः

नेत्रत्वक्नखपीतत्वं तृष्णास्तिक्तास्यता तथा ॥७० ॥

शुष्ककासोपपत्तिश्च लिंगं शीतज्वरस्य तु ॥

Sitakampa (tremors associated with cold), bhrama (vertigo), romaharasha (goose bumps), jrmbha (yawning) sirashula (pain in thehead) kati parshva shula, yellow coloration of eyes, klama (tiredness without exertion), bitter taste in the mouth, dry cough are the characteristics of sita jwara.

Notes: *Author has named this jwara as sitajwara and the symptoms mostly similar to vishamajawara of vata origin mentioned in Caraka.*

Doṣahetuka Jwara Lakṣaṇa:

शरीरं शीतलं यस्मिन्दाहतापौ करे पदि ॥ ७१ ॥ स्वरस्तु दुर्बलः पित्तप्रकोपो जायते ज्वरे ॥ ज्ञानाज्ञानक्रियाजन्यदोषहेतुक उच्यते ॥ ७२

This jwara is characterized by coldness in the body, burning sensation in the hands and feet and weakness in voice. It is to be noted that author mentions this doshahetuka jwara is the result of Jnanajnana Kriyarupa dosa. It means that this jwara is produced beacause of doing things knowingly or unknowingly.

Notes:

Ayurveda envisages three important causes of the disease. One among them is prajnaparadha, which indicates that the person indulges in activities though knows that particular activity causes disease. Probably above said jananajnana kriya rupa dosha concept similar to prajnaparadha.

Antardaha Jwara: The symptoms have taken from charaka chikista 3rd chapter under the name antarvega Jwara, but he has omitted bahirvega Jwara for the reasons not known.

Notes:

Antarvega Jwara means fever in which the symptoms are manifested internally and temperature cannot be felt. Symptoms of this fever include –

Antardaha – burning sensation inside the body; Adhika trshna – excessive thirst etc. Bahirvega jwara is characterized by excessive temperature in the exterior parts of the body and mildness of thirst etc. and it is curable.

Viṣamaśīta Jwara Lakṣaṇa:

आदौ मध्ये तथान्ते च मध्येऽन्ते वा प्रकुप्यति ॥ ७४ ॥

This is new jwara mentioned by the author .Its salient feature is occuring of fever, bhrama (vertigo), murcha (syncope), kampa (tremor) and also increase of tamoguna (feeling of darkness) which takes place in primary, middle and last stages of fever, this visama sitajwara can be made into curable condition by giving long term treatment.

Ama Jwara Lakṣaṇa

हल्लसस्तम्भस्त्वगुर्व्यरोचकम् । तंद्रालस्यविकारास्यवैरस्यगुरुगात्रता: ॥ ७६ ॥

क्षुतं च बहु मूत्रं च स्तब्धता बलवाञ्ज्वरः । लालाप्रसेको

आमज्वरस्य लिंगानि न दद्यात्तत्र भेषजम् ॥ ७७ ॥

The above verse taken from Madhavanidana.

Author has a tendency that many a time either he adds up or alters the original verses or delets some of the portion of the original verses .

Agantuka Aṣta Jwara

ग्रहावेशौषधविषक्रोधभीशोककामजः । अभिचारोद्भवश्चैव ह्यष्टरूपो ज्वरःस्मृतः ॥७८॥तंत्राभिचारकैर्मंत्रैर्जायते यस्य वै ज्वरः ॥८२॥ मोहो मूर्छा च तृष्णा स्यात् स्फोटकं जायते तथा

Author explains eight types of agantuka Jwara such as grahavesa aushadhaja, Vishaja, krodhaja, bhayaja, sokaja and kamaja. He did not follow the four type classification i.e. Abhighata, Abhichara, Abhishanga and Abhisapa mentioned in brihatrayee. He did not mention abhishanga and abhisapa types of abhighata Jwara.

Notes:

According to Brihatrayee Agantuj (which is cause by external factors) is of 4 varieties Viz,

Abhighataja – due to external injury

Abhishangaja – due to excess lust, anger, grief, poison, etc

Abhicharaja – Due to evil tantric rituals

Abhishapaja – due to Shapa (curse) of elderly

Saptavidha dosha (Jwara Doṣotpatti) :

अथ सप्तविधा दोषा वक्ष्यंते शास्त्रनिश्चिताः ॥ ८३ ॥ तरुण ज्वरमध्ये तु ह्यपथ्यजनितास्तथा । पटूवम्लतिक्तकटुककषायस्वादुभोजनात् । जलपानेन

शीतेन जलपानेन शीतेन वनितासंगमादुषः । । ८४॥ व्यायामचिंता शोकैश्च
ज्वरे दोषसमुद्भवः ॥

Person who indulges in improper dietary regimen of dosa develops saptavidha dosa, an exclusive contribution by the author.

Maha Dosha: Mahadosha get produced if the person afflicted with taruna Jwara indulges in food rich in tikta, katu, kashaya rasa, alcohol, water, cool habitat, and also indulging in sex, anger, walking long distances, who undergoes grief and worry.

Jwara Parivarjaneeya: As per Vaidyachintamani patient suffering from Jwara should avoid or not resort to adorning of flowers applying chandana, viewing moon, red clothes, ghrita, guda, gingelly oil, flavoured rice, cotton bed, new clothes, living in room with heavy breeze and contact of ladies.

Apathya dosha: Author explains general characteristics of apathya (substance which are not conducive to health).

तंद्रा मूर्छा भ्रमो दाहः प्रलापो हृदि वेदना ॥८७॥ अपथ्य दोषा विज्ञेया वैद्यविद्या विशारदैः Tandra (drowsiness), Murcha (syncope), bhrama (vertigo), daha (burning senasation) pralapa (delirium) hridaya vedana (angina pectoris) occurs because of apathya.

Stree Sangam dosha:

तरुणज्वरमध्ये च युवत्याः संगमो यदि ॥ ८८

जायते दारुणो दोषो हांगवैकल्यकंपने। वक्षोंतरे च संतापः प्रलापो दाहविभ्रमौ
॥ ८९ ॥

पाणिपादतले शैत्यं दोषः स्त्रीसंगजः स्मृतः ॥

The person who indulges in sex during febrile illness will have shivering, coolness of hand and feet etc.

Vishama dosa lakshana:

तृष्णा ज्वरश्च संतापः नाडीकुटिलवेगिनी ।। ९० ।। अंतर्दाहो मदो मूर्छा लिंगं विषमदोषके

The pulse will be crooked (kutila) and runs fast. Burning sensation of the stomach fever, fainting and intoxication are the symptoms.

Vishamaseeta dosha lakshana:

दिने द्वित्रिचतुर्वारं मुहुः शीतं मुहुज्वरः ।। ९१ ।।

दाहो मोहशिरोरुक्च जिह्वाकठिनकंटका । दोषं विषमशीतं च जानीयुर्वैद्यपारगाः ।। ९२

The patient will have fever with rigors and subsiding twice a day, thrice a day or four times a day. Another important symptom described by him is Jihwa Krathina Kantaka (A thorn like hardness in the tongue).

Notes: *Vishama means irregular. Dosha when attain vishama (state of increase or decrease resulting in the pathogenesis) cause disease.*

Pathological conditions of jihwa (tongue):

जिह्वा सरक्तवर्णा सकंटका द्रवसंयुता। ज्वरस्तृष्णा विदाहश्च रक्तजिह्वकलक्षणम् ।। ९३

जिह्वा पीता स्फुटच्छुष्का कंटकाढ्या ज्वरो भ्रमः । मदो मूर्छा गद्गदं च पीतजिह्वकलक्षणम् ।।९४।।कृष्णाजिह्वासुकठिना कंटकाढ्या ज्वरो भ्रमः । श्वासः कंडूर्मदस्तृष्णा स्याद्दोषः कृष्णजिह्वकः ।। ९५ ।।

एतेषां सप्तदोषाणां प्रमाणं चार्धमासकम् ।। ९७।।

अथवा सप्तदिवसं विज्ञेयं शास्त्रपारगैः ॥ Like this above mentioned seven Dosas duration will be 15 days to 7 days.

We find description of different kinds of clinical conditions pertaining to Jihwa (tongue) many a time. They include Raktajihwa, peetajihwa, Krishna jihwa, sweta jihwa (colour of tongue will be red, yellow, black and white respectiviely). In almost all jwaras we find that the mention of the disorders of jihwa such as the tongue feels hard, dry and thorny etc. This kind of vivid description about tongue is not to be seen in othertexts.

Jwara dinacharya:

अथ ज्वरदिने चर्या वक्ष्यते शास्त्रसम्मता ॥ ९८ ॥

ज्वरस्यादि दिने कुर्याल्लंघनं च ततः परम् ।

द्वितीयेऽहनि चोत्तिष्ठन् कुर्याद्द्विः दंतधावनम् ॥ ९९ ॥

जिह्वानिर्लेखनं कृत्वा क्षालयेदुष्णवारिणा ।

मूर्धिनर्वस्त्रं ततो बध्वा शयनं वामभागतः ॥ १०० ॥

पूर्ववल्लंघनं कुर्यात्तृतीये दिवसे ततः । चतुर्भागावशेषं तु ह्युष्णतोयं क्वचित्पिबेत् ॥ १०१ ॥ तत्तोयदोषनाशार्थमद्यात्कतकबीजकम् । चतुर्थे दिवसे प्राप्ते पूर्ववल्लंघनं चरेत् ॥ १०२ ॥

पंचमेऽहनि संप्राप्ते यवागूप्राशनं ततः । षष्ठेऽहनि तथा कुर्यात् प्रातर्वै सप्तमेहनि ॥ १०३ ॥

गंडूषं पूर्ववत्कृता ह्यौषधं संपिबेत्ततः । यवागूं पूर्ववत्प्राश्य ह्यौषधं त्रिदिनं पिबेत् ॥ १०४ ॥

जिह्वा पीता स्फुटच्छुष्का कंटकाढ्या ज्वरो भ्रमः । मदो मूर्छा गद्गदं च पीतजिह्वकलक्षणम् ॥१४॥

लंघनं चोष्णपानीयं लंघनं परमौषधम् ॥ लंघनं त्रिविधं प्रोक्तं कफे पित्तेऽनिले
क्रमात् । लंघनं चोपवासः स्याल्लंघनं भोजनं लघु ।। १०९ ।।

While describing about Jwara dinacharya author instructs following procedures in general to be followed by all the patients of fever. They are

Langhana at the onset of fever. On the 2nd day dantadhawana, cleaning of the tongue, and gargling with hot water. Afterwards a cloth is tied to the head and his left hand should be kept underneath the head and sleep the whole day without taking meal.

On third day langhana is to be continued and should only drink warm water boiled to 1/4th of its quanity. To get rid of doshas pertaining to water, he should take the gandha of kataka beejakam. Fourth day he should undergo fasting. Yavagu is to be taken on the fifth day and the same is to be followed on sixth day. On seventh day medicine is to be taken after gandhusha (gargling) then followed by yavagu. This procedure has to be followed for 3 days. One should take aushada (medicine) alone on ninth day, the fever gets subsided. During convalescence light food is advocated later virechankarma is advised.

The above said procedures are simple and easily adoptable, cost effectiveness makes it a praiseworthy contribution by the author.

Duration of jwara:

अतः परं प्रवक्ष्यामि ज्वरवारप्रमाणकम् । सप्तरात्रं वातिके च षडरात्रं पैत्तिके
ज्वरे ।। १०६ ।। नवरात्रं श्लैष्मिके च द्वंदजे दशरात्रकम् । ज्वरपाको भवेद्यत्र
ह्यत ऊर्ध्वज्वरं हरेत् ।। १०७ ।।

Author also mentions duration of jwara such as vatajwara is 7 days, pittajwara 6 days, kaphajwara 9 days and dwandwaja jwara will be for 10 days. After these stipulated periods jwara paka will take place and fever comes to normalcy.

Time of administration of gruel:

Author opines that for vata patients rice gruel should be given in the evening, early morning for pittajwara patient, whereas in afternoon for sleshmajawara patient rice gruel is to be given.

Author has omitted prakrita, vaikrita Jwara and also Jwaras of rtu as mentioned in brihatrayee probably due to its impractibility or difficult in identifying them.

Clarifying about langhana author says that fasting itself is langhana for vata, laghu bhojana for pitta Jwara, and ushnodaka for sleshma Jwara patients.

Maha Jwara: In Vaidya chintamani, the author has given elaborative description of this Jwara. Author has mentioned other new Jwara exclusively mentioned by him are given below stand as testimony for his significant knowledge about symptoms and disease especially for jwara. Under each jwara we find aggravation period of fever and instructed when to start treatment etc.

The following are the characteristics features.

Vata Jwara Lakshana: Important features are as follows:

This Jwara occurs because of sin of prajapeedana (harassing people).

This fever stays for 12 days continuously.

Since the first five days of the fever will be under aggravation. Hence he advises to treat the case after five days. Medicines such as pippalee churnam along with honey, Veeravikramarasa, vatagajankusa are prescribed. This jwara characterized by pain in the fore head, pain in the eye brows and pain in the eyes.

Paitya Jwara Lakshanams: The term paitya has been used to denote pitta Jwara.

Salient Features: Apart from the general symptoms, Jwara, Daruna daha, Bahu vedana etc are the important symptoms.

This fever also results due to praja peedana and suffers the patient continuously for ten days.

Prescription: Lavanga and Jeera mixed in sindhuram or veeravikramarasa for five days are prescribed.

Sleshma Jwara Lakshnas:

Apart from general symptoms we find symptoms like Jadatvam Sarvagatrana Sarva sandhishu Shula (rigidity and pain all over the joints). This fever is also results due to praja peedana in previous birth.

This fever suffers the patient for 12 days. The first seven days the fever is under tarunavastha (incubation period). Powder of trikatu added with lavanga along with honey is prescribed not only for this fever but also for many fevers which have been mentioned by him.

Veeravikramarasam or sindhuram or vatagatankusa administered to cure the disease.

Vata Paitya Jwara Lakshanas: Important symptoms include Bahu bhashanam (excessive talk), pralapam (delirium) and Daruna Shirashula (severe headache). This fever also results due to great sin of public harassment. This fever suffers the patient for sixteen days and will be under tarunavastha (immature state) for eight days. He prescribes granthikam (modi), devakusumam (Pippalimulam), magadham (lavanga) powder along with honey. Maha Lankeswararasam, Jogirasam is advised four times a day for 3 days.

Vata sleshma Jwara Lakhsanas (characteristics):

The main symptoms include Sarvanga sithilata (lassitude), severe pain in the head and eyes. The word Kapala has been used for Siras (head). Immature period is 3 days.

Notes:

In the above said fevers we find that he could precisely mentions for how many days the immature period lasts in each type of fever. He advises not to give any medicine during aggravation period. He prescribes rasoushadhas based on his experience in combating individual fevers. Veeravikramaras and Maha Jogirasa are generally indicated. We find public harassment as the cause for disease. The terms paitya (pitta) and daruna, maha indicate seriousness of a given condition. This are generally spoken by telugu people of southern region, it.

Paitya Sleshma Jwara: Important symptoms of this fever include daruna Jwara (dreadful fever). Kantaka Jihwitam (thorny tongue), Kaphodhriti (excessive phelghm formation) excessive sweating. This fever also results from harassing public. Taruna stage for 3 days. Trikatu, Jeera and Lavanga along with honey, and Vatagajankusa and sudarshanaras are the rasoushadhas used to treat this fever.

Vatapaitya Sleshma Jwara: karna nada (Tinnitus) and kapala (cephalus) a peculiar symptom used. Continuous sweating in hands, feet and the throat region are other symptoms mentioned.

Due to sin of public harassment in the previous birth mentioned as a cause of disease. For this he prescribes Varuna bark powder, Trikatu and Lavanga powdered and taken along with honey.

Rasoushadhas used are sudarshanarasam and Jogirasam etc.

Bhutavesa Jwaram characteristics: Author mentions peculiar symptoms such as Redness of eyes, face and severe warmth. It results due to public harassment (Prajapeedana). This fever's peculiarity is that it will always be under aggravation. Advocates trikatu, Jeerakam, Pippallu churna as anupana added with dhurjatirasa, Jogeerasa administered twice a day (ie prataha, Sayankala) (Timings of administering medicine is similar to modern parlance.).

Notes: *Prakruta Jwara are fevers manifesting in a season usually produced due to the aggravation of particular dosha during the season. On the contrary and Vaikruta Jwara is the fever manifesting in a season by dosha which is not normal for such dosha to have aggravation in that* season. Fevers manifesting due to spell or magic done by people who have attained perfection and success in these maneuvers are called as abhicharaja jwara. In bhutabhishangaja jwara, the fever would manifest with the symptoms of the same evil spirit, which has afflicted the person.

Abhicara jwara :

शिराभाराश्शरः कपस्सुस्निहानिः पिपासुता । रक्ताक्षितोयं स्रवति
पूर्वजन्मकृतात्तथा ॥ १४९ ॥ प्रजापीडनपापाच्च ह्यभिचारज्वरोद्भवे । तारुण्यं
द्विदिनं नित्यं ज्वरादौ दीयते रसः ॥ १५० ॥ शारिवादिव्यपुष्पं च मागधी
माक्षिकं यदि । गंधर्व रसनामा च जोगीरामसमाह्वयः ॥ १५१ ॥ अभिचारज्वरं
हन्तिं ह्यायुरारोग्यवर्धनः ॥

The important symptoms of Abhichara jwara are Hikka, hrillasa, jwara,, pralapa, kantakajihwa and jihwa shuskata (dryness of the tongue) . This jwara will be taruna for 2 days. In the primary stage sariba, lavanga, pippali with madhu is to be administred along with gandharva rasa or jogirasa.

Daiva prakopajwara:

ज्वरशीतं शिरोभारस्वेदसर्वांगशीतलम् ॥ १५२ ॥

हिध्मा हिक्का शिरःकंपो जडत्वं शूलमुत्कटम् । मूर्छा शोषश्श्रमश्चैव तंद्राश्वासः
कफस्तथा ॥ १५३॥ हीनस्वरस्सुत्पिनाशो मंदाग्निर्मलबन्धकः । उद्गारो वमनं
रक्तनेत्राद्वैतोयनिस्रुतिः ॥ १५४॥ पूर्वपापवशाच्चैव जायते
दारुणज्वरः।दैवप्रकोपनामाख्यस्तरुणं तं त्यजेन्नरः ॥ १५५॥ द्विकालं जीरकं
व्योषं वरालं माक्षिकं तथा । वैष्णवीरसमालिह्याज्जोगिनीरसमुत्तमम् ॥ १५६ ।
। दैवप्रकोपनामायं ज्वरः शाम्यति दारुणः

Jwara, sarvanga gaurava (heaviness of the body), jadatva (stiffness), tandra (drowsiness), hinaswara (feeble voice), netrasrava (lacrimation) raktavarna netra (redness of the eye) are some of the important symptoms. Jiraka and trikatu with madhu in the combination of vaishnavi jwara or jogirasa administered 2 times a day.

Bhiti (fear) jwara lakshana:

., रउत्पन्ने प्रलापो बहुभाषिता ।। १५७ ।।

तंद्रा स्वेदो महांस्तापो रक्तादृक्सत्त्वहीनता । शिरोक्षिवेदना कंपो दुर्भाषा भुक्तिवांच्छितम् ॥ १५८ ॥ सुप्तिहानिः शिरोभ्रंशः श्वासश्लेष्मासुशूलकम् । सर्वांगं शिथिलं शीतं रोमहर्षणशीतलम् ॥ १५९ ॥ दाहो हृदयमध्ये तु पिटकादंतमूलयोः । प्रजापीडनपापाच्च भीतिज्वरसमुद्भवः ॥ १६० ॥ तारुण्यं त्रिदिनं चादौ प्रयुंज्यादिमौषधम् । ग्रंथिकं दीप्यकं पुष्पमुमामहेश्वरो रसः ।। १६१ ॥ जोगीरससमायुक्तः माक्षिकं मागधीऽविषा । भीतिज्वरं चाशु हंति जीवेद्वर्षशतं नरः ।

Tivra jwara, bahu bhashana (excess of talk), adhika santapa (excess of hotness), rakta varna netra (reddish colour of eye), swasa, shiro bhramsa, sarvanga shithilata, etc., are important symptoms. This jwara will be in immature state for three days. Lavanga churna, ativisa, pippali administered in combination with umamaheswararasa and jogirasa.

Pisaca jwara lakshana

रक्ताक्षिदंतवदनं दुर्भाषा बहुभाषणम् । दाहमोहपिपासार्तिहूत्कारादारुणो ज्वरः ।। १६३॥ सर्वांगे मूर्ध्निकंपश्च भुक्ताविच्छा ह्याहर्निशम् । रोदनं वमनं हिक्का कासः श्वासश्च शीतलम् ॥ १६४॥ पिशाचज्वरसंभवे

Raktavarna netra, danta, mukha (red discolouration of eyes, teeth, and face) anucita bhashana (irrelevant talk), adhika bhashana (prattling), moha, hrillasa, sarvanga kampa (tremors all over the body), urdhwanga kampa rodana and possess sukshma nadi (slow pulse) . In this jwara fine powder made up of varuna, dhanyaka pippali, madhu administered in combination with Bhupati rasa or sindhura rasa. During taruna jwara no treatment is to be given but dhupa to be given made up of vana tulasi etc., given three times a day and also garudadyanjana to be applied to the eyes.

Gandharva jwara lakshana:

Sarvanga sopha (swelling all over the body), satva hinata (lacking moral courage), sithilata (lassitude) netra srava (lacrymation), pita varna (yellowish discolouration), bahumutrata are the characteristic features. During taruna jwara treatment should not be done. After this period powder of sariba, dhanyaka, lavanga pippali and ativisa should be administered in combination either of bhupati rasa, rasa sindhura, jogirasa If responds to this treatment the patient will live for hundred years .

Other important jwaras mentioned by him are

Sweda jwara:

श्वासोमूर्छाश्रमश्चैव जिह्वा कंटकिता मृदुः । वैरूप्यं वेदना कार्यं नाडी सूक्ष्मातिवेगता ।। १९८ ।। ज्वरः स्वेदो महाशीतं शीतलं बहुभाषणम् । दुर्भाषा ह्यतितंद्रा च हीनस्वरशिरोभ्रमौ ।। १९७ ।।

हिमाहिक्का तथोद्गारः शोफः कर्णकपालके । आननं करपादं च पीतवर्णं शिरोव्यधा ।। १९९ ।।

पूर्वपापात् प्रजाक्षोभात्स्वेदज्वरसमुद्भवे । त्रिदिनं वाथ चत्वारि पंच षड्वादिनानि च ।। २०० ।। व्योषं ग्रंथिकधान्ये च वरालमथ शारिवा । वरुणा त्वक् च दीयेत माक्षिकं चाद्रकद्रवः ।। २०१ ।।

सुवर्णभूपतिश्चैव रसो वातगजांकुशः । वीरविक्रमनामा च स्वेदज्वरनिवारकः ।। २०२ ।

Jwara, sweating, bahu bhashana (speaking in excess) durbhasha (prattling), atitandra (excessive dowsiness) swasa, murcha etc. jihwa mrudutva and kantaka (tender tongue and thorny) sopha in karna and kapala (swelling of ear and skull region), pita varna in mukha hasta pada (yellowish discolouration face, hands and feet) are the important symptoms, Sunthi, pipali, marica dhanyaka are to be administered along with bhupati, vatagajankusa, vira vikramaras (any one). This should be administered either 3 days or 4 days or 6 days in order to cure sweda jwara.

Krimijwara lakshana:

ज्वरश्च दारुणशूलमुन्नतोदरगौरवम् । उद्गारश्च तथा श्वासस्स्वेदसर्वांगशीतलम्
॥ २०३ ॥

It is characterized by daruna jwara, pain expansion of abdomen falling worms in vomiting daily, twenty thirty, hundred worms will come out. Anaha (distention above the pubic area) due to obstruction of urine and stools are the characteristic of krimi jwara. No treatment should be given in taruna jwara. Fine powder of jharsi, kadalikshara, vidanga trikatu, rasna, snuhi, sariba madhu mixed with talakeswararasa or suta sindhurarasa are to be administered twice daily for five days.

Haridra jwara:

ज्वरशीतं जडत्वं च सर्वांगं पीतवर्णकम् ॥ २०८ ॥

रक्तहीनं नखं नेत्रं शूलं संधिषु शोथकः । हिध्मा हिक्का तथोद्गारः
करपादं च शीतलं ॥ २०९ ॥

शिरोवातशिरोभ्रंशो जिह्वावदनतिक्तता । पिपासा कंठशोषश्च
हृत्तापश्चाग्निमांद्यकम् ॥ २१० ॥

मलबंधो मले शोषोप्यरुचिश्लेष्मणः सदा । निष्ठ्यूतिः फेनिलं वक्त्रं
तापश्च बहुभाषणम् ॥ २११॥

प्रजापीडनपापेन हरिद्राज्वरसंभवे । तारुण्ये शून्यतां याते चत्वारि
दिवासानि वै ॥ २१२ ॥ वरालं शारिवा धान्यं माक्षिकं धूर्जटीरसः ।
जोगीरसो वैष्णवाख्यस्सुदर्शनरसो हितः ॥ २१३॥

हरिद्राज्वर नाशाय नात्रकार्या विचारणा ।

Important symptoms being fever, stiffness yellowish colouration in all parts of the body. Foamness in the mouth, dryness of the stool. Similar to other jwara powder of sariba, dhanyaka is to be given with madhu followed by administration of dhurjati rasa, jogirasa, vaishnavi rasa, sudarsana rasa for a period of 4 days.

ज्वरो गंभीरसंतापः कंठे लिंगे भ्रुवोर्द्वये ॥ २१४॥

नाभिमूले हृदस्थाने स्तनमूले ललाटके । विदाहोऽरतिचिंते च नाडीवेगो
बलाधिकः ॥ २१५॥

पिपासा च शिरोभ्रंशस्त्वन्नकांक्षा मुहुर्मुहुः । मानसीरतिकांक्षा च
मंदहासोऽहानिद्रता ॥ २१६ ॥ प्रजापीडनपापेन कामज्वरसमुद्भवे।
द्विकालं चंदनं लेप्यं महाराजमृगांककम् ॥ २१७॥ चिंतामणिरसं
दद्याद्द्राक्षाखर्जूरमिश्रितम् । तरुण्ये शून्यतां याते कामज्वरनिवृत्तये ॥
२१८॥

Jwara and santapa (incread temperatue, hot blushes) constantly thinking about coitus, rapid pulse, anidra (insomnia) are the main features of Kama jwara. Treatment includes lepa (application) with the fine powder of chandana and administered along with maharaja mrigankarasa, cintamani rasa with draksha and kharjura .

Several jwaras have been named by the author basing on the period of time in the day or onset of fever Eg., pratah kala jwara (fever occuring during the period of sun rise). Jihva tiktata, mukha tiktata, karapada sitalata (cold hands and feet) are some of the important features of this fever. Likewise in madhyama jwara, jwara, bahu bhashanam, bahumutrata (polyuria) are the important features. Fine powder of pippali along with suta sindura or jogirasa administered after langhana.

In Sayankala jwara the person will feel very cold in the evening, and suffers from jwara, jihwa tiktata, tikta (bitterness of the mouth). Both madhyama jwara and sayankala jwara considered being the result of prajapidana papa. Both madhyahna jwara and sayankala jwara share similar line of treatment.

Sosa jwara lakshana: Sosa (cachexia), santapa (hot feel), murcha (syncope), severe pain, feeling of coldness in the body frequent micturition, presence of thorn like structures on the tongue are some of the characteristic features. Prajapidana (harrassing public) is considered as the cause for just like other jwaras. Lavanga powder, dhaniya given with vaishnavi ras, jogiras administered to cure this condition.

Vrana jwara

Painful ulcer, saithilyata, chittabhrama (unconsciousness) tikta jihwata (feeling bitterness of the tongue, kapalasosa (dryness of skull), karna sosa (dryness of ears). The fever is considered as purvajanmaja prajapidana papa (harassment people in previious birth). Treatment consists of pippali marica, lavanga churna in combination with either viravikrama rasa or vranantaka rasa which is administered 2 times a day.

Santapa jwara:

Santapa jwara occurs due to continuous exposure to sunlight, severe pain fever, burning sensation boils in tooth and gums, mukham kumkuma sadrusam (redness of the face similar to saffron) jihwa vadana madravam (dryness in the tongue and mouth), hridaya vedana (pain in the heart) and hasta pada kampa (tremors in hands and foot) . Bath with badari patra kashaya indicated. Treatment consists varuna mula along with sita (sugar candy) is to be administered along with dhurjati rasa, jogiras 2 times. Diet should consists of buttermilk and salidhanya .

Swara hina jwara: low rise of temperature. Hasta jadata (stiffness of the hands), pada jadata (stiffness of the foot) jihwa sosha, mukha sosha (dryness of the mouh), sarvanga sithilata (weakness in the body parts) are the important symptoms. Fever will be in immature stae for 1 day. Treatment is varuna churna, trikatu, lavanga administered in combination with maharaja mriganka rasa orchintamani rasa or jogirasa .

Abhighata jwara: Because of injury vata and sleshma get vitiated and produce abhightaja jwara (fever developed due to injury) . Important symptoms include jwara, satva hinata (lacking moral courage), loss of shine in the body, salivation, redness of eyes, dryness of tongue. If the patient of abhighataja jwara resorts to wearing of flowers, coitus, massage, bath etc would lead to complications. In this conditions dhurjati rasa, vaishnavi rasa jogirasa, twice a day recommended.

Ama jwara: Apart from the usual Jwara Symptoms stools consists with Ama, satvahinata (lack of mental strength), "Raktakshi Jihwa vadanam" (redness of eyes, tongue and mouth) and Akshitoyam, shula (Watering of the eye and severe pain in the eyes) are important. This jwara results due to sin of previous birth.

Powder of Jathiphalam, Jatipatram, Vriddhadarukam, ahiphenakam, lavanga added with honey and administered with the combination of sindhura, maliniras or grahani vajra kavataras to relieve one from amajwara.

Agnimandya Jwara:

अग्निमान्द्यज्वरे हीनं सत्वं कांतिविहीनता । मंदाग्निर्मलबन्धश्च ज्वरो दाहश्शिरोव्यथा ॥ २६७॥ कासश्श्वासश्च शुष्कांगमन्नद्वेषो ह्यरोचकम् । उद्गारो वमनं हिध्मा जिह्वावदनतिक्तता ॥ २६८॥ निर्वीर्यं मुखशोषश्च पाणिपादं सशूलकम् । पूर्वजन्मकृतात्पापादग्निमांद्यज्वरोद्भवः ॥ २६९॥ चतुर्दिनं द्विकालं च व्योषचूर्णं तथार्द्रकम् । भूपतिं रससिंदूरं रसं वातगजांकुशम् ॥ २७० ॥ । सेवयेद्बुद्धिमन्वैद्यो ह्यग्निमांद्यज्वरापहम्

This is another newly mentioned clinical condition with respect to jwara .In this we find special symptoms like satvahinata (loss of mental courage), kantihinata (Loss of glow), sushkangata (dryness of the body) etc. He advises administering of digestant medicines like trikatu, ardraka swarasa in combination with bhupati rasa, rasa sindhura or vatagajankusa two times a day for four days .

Vamana jwara:

वमनज्वर आम्लं च तिक्तं वमति संवतम् ॥ २७१॥ Amla tikta vamanam (vomiting of sour substances), burning sensation of the heart. Vamana jwara, new jwara mentioned by the author. It's symptoms include, sarvanga saithilyam (debilitating illness of entire body), Satva hinata lacking moral courage), hastapada sitalata (coldness of hands and feet) . This Jwara also due to praja kshobha mahapapa (big sin) .For this jwara author prescribes panchamritarasa, parpatirasam with honey as anupana advised twice a day for four months.

Hidhma Jwara:

The following are the special symptoms mentioned such as Hidhma (hiccups), Seetala Sarvangam (cold clad skin), Vamanam tiktamlakam (vomiting of bitter and sour material) . Kapaladaha (burning sensation of the head), Karna daha (Burning sensation of the ear), nasa daha (burning sensation of the nose) sosha (severe tissue depletion), Pitakam danta bandhakam (boils in the gums), sirobhramsam (hanging of the head), heenaswaram (feeble voice) etc. Advises durgrahasya churnam (fagonia Arabica) with madhu as anupana. Vaishna Veerasam, Jogeerasam is advised twice a day relieves one from hidma Jwara, and also lives for hundred years .

Hikka Jwara:

निस्सत्वता वमिश्वासः प्रलापश्चातिसारकः । सुम्लिहानिशिरोभारी
हत्तापस्संधिशूलकम् ॥ २८२॥ प्रजापीडनपपाच्च हिक्काज्वरसमुद्भवे ।
ज्वरादौ नास्ति तारुण्यं द्विकालं व्योषधान्यकम् ॥ २८३ ॥ ग्रंथिकं
शिखरीबीजचूर्णं कार्पासचूर्णकम् । सिंदूरं वैष्णवीसूतं जोगीरस समाह्वयम् ॥
२८४॥हिक्काज्वरे ददेत्तीव्रं जीवेद्वर्षशतं नरः ।

In this jwara unique symptoms like hikka (hiccups), mandagni (loss of digestive fire), Hridaya tapam, Sandhishula etc, are produced because of praja peedana mahapapa (public harassment) . Sindhuram or Vaishnaveerasam or Jogirasam taken along with powder consisting of Trikatu, Pippaleemulam, Sikharee beeja churnam, karpasa (gossypium herbaceum) as anupana advocated to relieve from the disease.

Notes:

Both Hidma and Hikka are considered as synonyms, but here author depicted them as two separate clinical conditions.

In many of the formulations we find this tag sentence i.e "Jeevedavarshasatam" (lives for hundred years) as tag line.

Anidra Jwara:

अनिद्राज्वरसंतापतृष्णामोहश्रमभ्रमाः ॥ २८५॥

जिह्वावदनशोषश्च श्वासश्शीतलगात्रता । प्रलापो बहुपित्तं च जानुजंघातिवेदना ॥ २८६ ॥ हीनस्वरःसदा कासमूर्छाशोषशिरोभ्रमाः । पूर्वपापानुसाराच्च ह्यनिद्राज्वरसंभवे ॥ २८७॥ द्विकालं ग्रंथिकं धान्यं वरालं व्योषशारिवाः । सुदर्शनं धुर्जटिं च स्वर्णभूपतिमाददेत् ॥ २८८ ॥ अनिद्रा ज्वरनाशाय ह्यायुर्वृद्धिर्भवेत् सदा ॥

Another peculiar Jwara mentioned by the author is Anidra (loss of sleep) Jwara. The main symptoms include Anidra, Jwara, Santapa, moha, srama (fatigue), bhrama, etc. Bahupittam (The term exclusively used by him, means excess of pitta) Results due to sin of previous birth. To subside this fever author advises Sudarshanarasam, dhurjatirasam, suvarnabhupatirasam taken along with powder of lavanga with Trikatu as anupana.

Kasa jwara:

ज्वरः कासः पिपासा च ष्ठीवनं रक्तफेनिलम् ॥ २८९ ॥

उद्गारो वमनं तंद्रा शिरोभ्रमणकंपने ॥ २९०। निस्सत्वं स्वरहानिश्च नादः कर्णकपालके । कुक्षिशूलं चातिसारो हिध्मा हिक्का ह्यनिद्रता ॥ २९९ ।.
अतिरक्तमतिश्वेतं मूर्छाश्वासश्रमभ्रमाः ।

Another peculiar Jwara mentioned by him is kasa Jwara. The important symptoms include Jwara, Steevanam raktaphenilam (expectoration of white or red coloured sputum), sirobhramanam (vertigo), Kampanam, Nissatvam (lassitude), and Karna kapalanadam (kapala nadam not mentioned in any ayurvedic text it indicates revolving sound in ears and skull.) .

Interestingly in this fever the symptom kasa is not mentioned . Many a time the term kasa used to describe respiratory affectations.

Prescriptions: Umamaheswararasam, Jogeerasam, Bhupathirasam used along with powder of (varalam) lavanga, sariba, varuna to relieve from Kasa Jwara.

DhatugataJwara: Symptoms mentioned in Vaidya chintamani are totally different from those mentioned in Madhavanidana and other ayurvedic texts. These Dhatugata jwara considered are due to sin of harassment of public in previous birth as the sole cause for the development of dhatugata Jwara. The following are some of the salient features with respect to dhatu gata jwara are quite unique of him. They are as follows

Rasa gata jwara lakshanas :

Prior to manifesting of fever in the body rasa dhatu gata jwara will occur. Jwara, siro gaurava (heaviness of the head), feeble voice, sweating over the throat dryness of the tongue, weakness of mental faculty are the major features.

Pippalimula churnam, ativisa along with umamaheswara rasa, swarana bhupati rasa, jogirasa two times a day.

Rakta gata jwara lakshana:

Main features of this jwara include Sweda, bhrama, siro bhrama, atisara burning sensation of the hands and foot, blood in stools, feeling of loosness and fatigue in the body parts .Treatment consists of administering sariba, trikatu, vaca, dhanyaka churna and madhu along with dhurjati rasa, or gandharva rasa or jogirasa .

Mamsagata jwara:

Fever that existing in rasadhatu if exceeds 7 nights enters rakta dhatu, and if raktasrita Jwara exceeds 25 days then enters mamsa. Then it continues upto 2/1/2 months. It is characterized by feeling of cold hiccup, flatulence, and vomitings, bitterness in tongue and mouth and feeble voice. Author advises Lakshmi vilasa rasa, pancamrita rasa, sindhura are to be administered twice a day.

Medogata jwara:

After the completion of 2 months jwara converts to medo gata jwara .It is characterized by headache, giddiness, thirst, dyspepsia, suskata (dryness of the body) .

Treatment: Gajagandharasayana, panchamrita rasayana, mandura, parpati, kravyada rasa are to be administered depending on the condition upto 4 months. If medo gata jwara not treated in 5 months the jwara turns into astigata jwara.

Astigata jwara: Impotant symptoms are continuous fever, antardaha (burning sensation inside the body), emaciation, pandu varna (pale white colour), sira snayu asthi vedana (pain in the veins, ligaments and bones) and adhmana (flatulence).

Sukragata jwara: The symptoms are nidradhikyata, (excessive sleeping), pralapa (delirium), sajnanasa (loss of sensation). If these symptoms are persisting then it is considered incurable.

Visama jwara: Fluctuations in the body temperature, sudden occurrence of the severe fever, some times getting sleep and some times not. Some times fever recurs for 2 days and sometimes occurs for 4 days known as visama jwara (intermittent fever)

Murcha jwara: Severe fever among all fevers known as murcha jwara when patient becomes cold the patient develops tandra (drowsiness) and severity of jwara increases, if patient gets relief from jwara he also gets relief from murcha (syncope). This murcha jwara occurs at the time of death.

Sita jwara: Sitakampa (tremors associated with cold, pain in the head, pelvic region, and lateral side of the body. tiredness without exertion (klama) thirst, bitter taste in the mouth etc, are the characteristics of sitajwara lakshanas.

Dosahetuka jwara:

Coldness of the body, hastapada daha (burning sensation of palms and foot). This jwara is produced because of doing things knowingly or unknowingly.

Antardaha jwara:

Antardaha (Heat interior of the body), atitrishna (excessof thirst), pain in asthi and sandhi (pain in bone and joints), loss of glow in the body are the characteristics.

Visama sita jwara: jwara, bhrama, kampa, feeling of darkness, occurs in primary, middle, and last stages of fever.

Ama jwara: The symptoms are, lalapraseka (dribbling of saliva), thickness of the skin, mukha vairasya (distaste of mouth), angagaurava (heaviness of the body), sneezing, bahumutrata (ploy uria), stabdata and severity of fever.

Agantuka asta jwara: Author classifies agantuka jwara into eight types. They are Grahavesa, Aushadha, visa, krodha, bhaya, soka, kama, and abhicara.

Grahavesa jwara lakshana:

Udvga (excitement) hasya (laughing), rodana (crying), guruta (heaviness)

Aushadhagandhaja jwara:

Murcha, sirashula, vamana, kshavathu (sneezing)

Visajwara akshanas:

Krishna varna of mukha (blackish discolouration, atisara (diarrhea), aruchi (distaste), trishna (thirst), toda (irritation due to itching) and murcha.

Krodha, bhaya, soka jwara lakshanas:

Kampa (shivering) will be produced in the jwara which is occurring because of bhaya soka, pralapa ad krodha.

Kama jwara lskhana: citta vibhrama, (associated with madness &preservation of mind, tandra (drowsiness) alasya (laziness), abhojana (not taking food) hridaya vedana (pain in the heart region), dryness in the body.

Abhicara jwra lakshana: Fever which occurs because of tantra, mantra will have moha (delusion), murcha, trishna and sphota (boil).

Pitaka Jwara:

ज्वरो दारुण संतापो दाहमोहशिरोभ्रमाः ॥ ३२७ ॥

श्वेतसर्षपतुल्यं च सर्वांगे पिटकोद्भवः । जिह्वावदनशुष्कत्व कंटके सुप्तिशून्यता ॥ ३२८ प्रलापो बहुभाषित्वं नेत्रयोर्वेदनोद्भवः । फूत्कारः फेनसंजुष्टस्वरहीनत्वं शीतले ॥ ३२९

सर्वांगकंपनं चैव जानुजंघातिवेदना । उद्गारो वमनं हिक्का पिटकाज्वरसंभवे ॥ ३३० त्यक्त्वा तरुणतां वैद्यो लंघनं वर्जयेद्बुधः । द्विकालं चतुरो वारान् द्राक्षाखर्जूरधान्यकम् ॥ ३३१

व्योषं वरालं कल्कं च धूर्जटीरसमिश्रितम् । जोगीरसं प्रयुज्जीत पिटकज्वर नाशकम्

Highriseof temperature, daha (burning sensation), moha (delirium), sirobhrama (vertigo) Sweta sarshapa tulya sarvange Pitaka (development white gingelly seed like boils).

Dhurjatiras, Jogirasa appears to be popular prescription in those days for being very efficacious hence prescribed frequently .Here the duration of treatment is limited to 4 days.

Sphotaka Jwara (vesicular eruptions):

दारुणो ज्वरतापश्च विलापो बहुवेदना । मुद्गबीजसमाश्चैव स्फोटका दाह उत्कटः ॥ ३३३ तथैव हृदिसन्तापस्तंद्राशोषः प्रलापकः । निस्सत्वं स्वरहीनत्वं श्वासश्चैव सवेदनः ॥३३४॥

कुक्षिशूलं चातिसरसूक्ष्मानाडीविवर्णता । हास्यं गीतं सुप्ती हानी रक्ताक्षरस्रावयेज्जलम् ॥ ३३५ ॥

पूर्वपापावशाच्चैव स्फोटकज्वरसंभवे । दिनमेकं चतुर्वारं वरालं धान्यजीरकम्
॥ ३३६ ॥ द्राक्षां दद्यादुष्णातोयं स्फोटकज्वरनाशकम् । तारुण्यं त्रिदिनं प्रोक्तं
पश्चादारोग्यसंभवः ॥

Here the eruptions are described equal to mudga beeja. In this fever nadi will be slow. It also results from sin of previous birth. To relieve this, Kalka of lavanga (syzygium aromaticum), dhaniya (coriandrum sativum), Jeeraka (cuminumcyminum), draksha (vitis vinifera) and ushnodaka (warm water) is advised to take four times a day. It is said that the fever lasts for 3 days and later subsides. Such statements reveal of their knowledge about the prognosis and self-limiting nature of the disease.

Apart from the general symptoms we find new descriptions like bheeshana jwara (high rise of temperature) kampa (tremor). Nadi will be slow but some times runs fast. The sputum appears like flour (nishtutihi pistavadbhaveth). Treatment comprises Churna of Varuna (crataeva nurvala) bark, lavanga, dhanyaka, chitramula are added to rasoushodhas like sudarshanaras, uma maheshwararas, maha jogi ras and administered to relieve the fever.

Sopha Jwara Lakshana:

Sopha means swelling or oedema.

ज्वरश्च दारुणश्शीतं शोफस्सर्वांगसंगतः । मूर्ध्नि चात्यंतशूलं च शोषः कर्णे
कपालके ॥ ३४४॥ निस्सत्वं वमनं हिध्मा रोमहर्षश्च जृंभणम् ।
प्रजापीडनपापच्च शोफज्वरसमुद्भवे ॥ ३४५ ॥ तारुण्यं पंचरात्रं स्यात्
त्रिकालं ग्रंथिकं वचाम् । व्योषं वह्निं मिशिं रास्नां गंधर्वरसमुत्तमम् ॥३४६॥
वातगजांकुशम् । सेवयेद्बुद्धिमन्वैद्यश्शोफज्वरनिबर्हणम् ॥ ३४७॥महाजोगीरसं
चैव चैव रसं

In this important symptoms include Tivra jwara (high rise of temperature), sarvanga sotha (Swelling all over the body) pida in urdhwa bhaga (pain in the upper portion of the body). Sosa in karna and kapala (dryness in ears and skull). The fever will be under aggravation for 5 days. After these 5 days treatment has to be started. This fever also said to be cured with gandharva rasa, mahajogirasam.

Notes: *Here we find medicine administered three times a day and with a prohibition not to use medicine for five days. Sopha synonym for sotha means oedema or swelling of the body.*

Anaha Jwaram:

आनाहो मलबन्धश्च मंदाग्निर्वलिशूलकम् । ज्वरशीतं शिरोभारः कर्णयोर्घोष उत्कटः ॥ ३४८॥ चापल्यं चंचलानाडी ह्यतिसूक्ष्मा च वेगिता । पिपासा कंठशोषश्च बलाहान्यंगभारके ॥ ३४९॥

पांडुवर्णश्च रक्ताक्षि सर्वदा रोमहर्षणम् । मूत्रं मुहुर्मुहुर्वेगात् वदनानाहजे ज्वरे ॥ ३५० ॥

लंघयेत्पंचरात्रं च ततः कुर्याच्चिकित्सितम् । त्रिकालं सेवयेत् स्तन्ये माक्षिकेव्योषणशिशरम् ॥ ३५१ ॥ । च रसभूपतिम् । उमामाहेश्वरं चैव धूर्जटिं रसमेव च ॥ ३५२ ॥ ।

सदर्शनरसं वैश्वानरं वैश्वानरं च आनाहज्वरनाशस्स्याजीवेद्वर्षशतं नरः

Author mentions peculiar symptoms like Karnayo dgosha utkataha (roaring noice in the ears), anaham (distension of the abdomen due to obstruction of urine and stools), Nadi will be fluctuant, some times it is slow and some times moves fast. Balahanya anga bharakam (weakness and feeling of heaviness). 5 days fasting is specifically indicatedin this fever. Later medicine has to be started. It is amazing to note that in some fevers he prescribes medicines and declares that the fever will get subside for sure and lives for 100 years.

Trikala Jwara:

प्रातः काले च मध्याह्ने सायाह्ने शीतावाञ्ज्वरः ॥ ३५३ ॥

प्रलापो दंतघट्टश्च हास्यं गीतं विरूपता । मुखं कुंकुमसंकाशं निस्सत्वं स्वरहीनता ॥ ३५४॥

तंद्राऽनिद्रा तथा दाहो जिह्वावदनकंटकम् । मूर्छा चातिश्रमश्चैव शोषाश्श्वासोऽधृतिस्तथा ॥ ३५५॥

हिक्का शोफः कर्णमूले ग्रहणीव्यापदेव च । प्रजापीडनपापाच्च त्रिकालज्वरसंभवे

Fever is associated with cold in trikala i.e in early morning, afternoon and evening. Mukham kumkuma sankasam (face becomes red like kumkum), mukha kanthaka (presence of thorns over the mouth), karna mula shotha (inflammation of the root of the ear), swarahinata (feeble voice). This fever will have tarunavastha for 4 days.

Advises Dhurjateerasam, parpatiras, ummaheshwararas in the aggravating period itself to relieve the disease.

Sannipata Jwara:

ज्वरो भीषणदाहश्च नाडी सूक्ष्मगतिस्तथा ॥ ३५९ ॥ स्वेदशीतं च सर्वांगे पिपासा कंठकंटकम् । हीनस्वरो बुद्धिहानिर्हास्यं दुर्भाषणं तथा ॥ ३६० ॥ स्वल्पश्रुतिः कर्णनादस्तंद्राघोपः कपालके । निस्सत्वमंगजडता सर्वसंधिषु मारुतः ॥ ३६१ ॥ रक्ताक्षि कांटकाजिह्वा मूर्छा शोषः श्रमस्तथा । शिरोभ्रमणशूलं च प्रलापः श्वासकासकौ ॥ ३६२ ॥

पूर्वपापानुसाराच्च सन्निपातज्वरोद्भवे । तारुण्यं चैकरात्रं स्याच्चतुर्वारं दिने दिने ॥ ३६३ ॥ आर्द्रकद्रवसंयुक्त उमामाहेश्वरो रसः ॥ ३६४॥

धूर्जटीरसको देयो रसो वातगजांकुशः । गंधर्वंरसयुक्तश्च सन्निपातज्वरापहः ॥ ३६५॥

Following are the important symptoms of sannipata jwara.

Bheeshana daha (excessive thirst); Kantaka Jihwa (thorning of tongue).

Swalpa Sruti (Hearing of sounds at lower phase), Buddhihani (loss of memory), durbhasa (irrelevant speech), sarvanga jadata (stiffness in the body), kantha jihwa (thorn like structures in the throat).

Sushka Jwara:

भीमज्वरो महातापशिरोदृग्वेदनाभ्रमः ॥ ३६९॥

शुष्कांगं शीतलं स्वेदः प्रलापो दन्तघट्टनम् । जडत्वं सर्वगात्राणामानाहश्चाग्निमांद्यकम् ॥ ३७० ॥ पुलकश्चर्मधात्वोश्च प्रलेपस्सुमिशून्यता । तंद्रैव गुणसंप्राप्तिर्दुर्भाषाक्रोधसंयुता ॥ ३७१ ॥ पूर्वपापानुसारेण शुष्कज्वरसमुद्भवे । तारुण्ये शून्यतां याते धूर्जटीरसमुत्तमम् ॥ ३७२॥ पंचामृतंपर्पटीं च ह्याश्वगंधादिचूर्णकम् । माक्षिकैर्मिश्रितं नित्यं सेवयेद्बुद्धिमान्भिषक् ॥ ३७३ ॥ शुष्कज्वरं हरेच्चैव जीवेद्वर्षशतं नरः ॥

Apart from general symptoms, important symptoms include Bheema Jwara (severe fever), Maha tapa (rise in body temperature), Durbhasha (Irrelevant talk). To relieve this Dhurjateerasam, panchamritarasam, parpateerasam, Aswagandhadi churnam along with honey is prescribed. Author says it relieves the fever in the aggravation period itself and the person lives for 100 years.

Ekahika Jwara:

ज्वरोऽतिदारुणश्चैव दाहो मोहशिरोव्यथा ॥ ३७४ ॥प्रलापो बहुदुर्भाषा ह्युद्दारो वमनं सदा । हिध्मा श्वासशिरोभ्रंशस्सत्वंहानिः पिपासुता ॥ ३७५ ॥

एकरात्रमतिक्रम्य सशीतज्वरसंभवः । पूर्वजन्मकृतात्पापादेतज्जवरसमुद्भवः ॥ ३७६ ॥ उपावासद्वयं कार्यमौषधं सेवयेदनु । वरालं ग्रंथिकं पत्रं जोगीरससुमूपती ॥ ३७७ ॥ वैष्णवी रसनामानमेकाह ज्वरशांतये ।

Apart from the usual Jwara symptoms we find some other important symptoms such as Bahudurbhasha (irrelevant talk/prattling).

Advises Lavanga churna, pippalimula, tejapatra with jogirasa bhupati rasa vaishnavi rasa for administration.
Fasting is done for 2 days, then medicines is administered.

Dwyahika Jwara:

ज्वरो रौद्रो महाशीतमतिक्रम्य द्विरात्रकं ॥ ३७८ ॥

दाहो मोहशिरोभारः पिपसा स्वेद उत्कटः । उद्गारो वमनं हिध्मा ह्रक्ष्णोश्च भ्रमवेदने ॥ ३७९॥ सन्तापः करपादे च सुमिहानिर्बलक्षयः । निष्ठ्यूतिः फेनयुक्ता च करपादं च शीतलम् ॥ ३८० ॥ पूर्वपापानुसाराच्च द्वाहिकज्वरसंभवः । तारुण्ये शून्यतां याते भूपतीरस उत्तमः ॥ ३८१ ॥

जोगीरसः प्रदातव्यो द्वयाहिकज्वरशांतये

High rise of temperature associated with sita, daha, moha etc. It occurs lapse of 2 days. In this we observe 2 types symptoms such as hasta pada santapa, and also hasta pada sita, phenayukta nishteevana (sputum associated with foam). In this fever author recommends medicines after the initial aggressive period gets under control.

Tryahika Jwara:

ज्वरो घोरो महाशीतमतिक्रम्य त्रिरात्रकम् ॥ ३८२ ॥ रोदनं कंपितं चांगं दाहो मोहश्श्रमस्तथा । निस्सत्वं शुष्कतांगानां नेत्रे तोयस्रवस्सदा ॥ ३८३ ॥ अरुचिश्चाग्निमान्द्यं च जडत्वं सर्वसंधिषु । अजीर्णारुचिविष्टभ भक्तद्वेषस्तथैव

च ॥ ३८४॥ श्वासः कफो महाशोषः पूर्वपापानुसारतः । त्र्याहिकज्वरउत्पन्ने जायन्ते नित्यदुःखदे ॥ ३८५ ॥ द्विजद्रव्यापहरणाच्चिरकालं च पीडयेत् । तारुण्यं चैकरात्रं स्याच्छीतभूपतिमिश्रतम् ॥ ३८६ ॥

गंधर्व रसनामानं माहाजोगीरसं तथा । माक्षिके सेवयेन्नित्यं त्रिरात्रज्वरनाशकम्
॥ ३८७ ॥

Most dreadful seeta Jwara (Jwaro ghoro maha seta mati kramya triratrakam) occurs after the lapse three days. This fever suffers the person continuously. In this also we find symptoms like tearing (lacrimation) of the eyes, vistambha (constipation) and annadwesha (Anorexia).

Chaturthika Jwara: Jwara coming on the fourth day. Sithilatha (weakness of body parts) pain in the upper portion of the body, jihwa sushkata (dryness of the tongue) vertigo (brama), Seetala Karapadam are the main symptoms . Prescription includes administering of jogirasa, bhupati rasa, and vaishnavi rasa.

Panchahika Jwara: Passing of five nights, the fever sets in with rigors. Important symptoms include angasushkata (cachexia), dryness of the body siropida (pain in the head), netra pida (eye pain), sotha (oedema), shoola and atisara (diarrhea) . For this, lakshminarayana, lauha panchamrita rasa, bhupati rasa, mahajogirasa are administered for 1 or 2 months.

Masanta Jwara:

मासांते च ज्वरशशीतं दाहस्सन्तापमूर्छिते ॥ ४०१॥शिरो भारशिरोभ्रंशश्श्वासश्श्लेष्माबलाल्पता । अजीर्णारुचिविष्टंभा अन्नद्वेषशिरोभ्रमः । । ४०२॥ अक्षिकर्णे च शूलं च पीनसो नेत्रवारि च । पूर्वपापानुसाराच्च मासांतज्वरसम्भवे ॥ ४०३॥ मासान्काकजंघाकषायके ।

धूर्जटीरसमादद्यात्पंचामृतरसं तथा । ।४०४।। द्विकालं चतुरो महाजोगीरसं चैव मासांतज्वरशांतये ।।

If the fever occurs after a lapse of one month period it is known as masanta jwara. Important symptoms include fainting, dyspnoea, siro bhara, siro bhramsa (hanging of the head), netra shula, karna shula, netra srava (discharge from nose). He prescribes kakajangha rasa, dhurjati rasa, maha jogirasa for four months..

Varshantika Jwara:

वर्षांते च भवेच्छीतं ज्वरो दाहशिरो व्यथा ।। ४०५ ।।कर्णे कपाले नासायां भृशं सागरघोषकः । शुष्कांगं सत्वहीनत्वं संधिशूलातिशोफकौ ।। ४०६ ।। अग्निमान्द्यमजीर्णत्वमन्नद्वेषो ह्यरोचकः । नेत्रं स्नवति तोयं च सप्तधातुषु शोषणम् ।।४०७।। जिह्वावदनतिक्तता । प्रजापीडनपापाच्च हिध्माशोषश्रमश्चैवद्विकालं पंचमासांश्च सुदर्शनरसायनम् । उमामाहेश्वरं सूतंमहाराजमृगांकचजोगीरससमायुम् । सेवयेद्बुद्धिमांश्चैव वत्सरज्वरसम्भवे ।।४०८।। पंचामृतसुपर्पटीम् ।। ४०९ ।। वर्षांतज्वरशान्तये ।। ४१०।।

Fever occurs after lapse of 1 year. Patient develops rigors fever, headache and develops sound like a roar of the sea. (Nasayam bhrisam sagara ghoshakaha). We find other peculiar symptoms like mukhatikta (bitterness of the mouth), jihwatiktata (bitter taste in the tongue).

He prescribes sudarashana rasa, umamaheshwara rasa, jogirasa to treat this condition.

Importance of diagnosis:

Author insists that the physician should learn the concepts of about the knowledge of medicine thoroughly, and once the proper diagnosis is made, then only the success of treatment is possible.

Kashaya:

After completion of jwara prakaranam author mentions about the preparation of kashayas to cure the aggravation of each of the dosha i.e vata, pitta, kapha. Later he mentions about, kashayas prepared to suit 2 doshas like vata sleshna pitta sleshma etc. After that we find kashayas mentioned which are prepared exclusively targeting to cure specific jwaras and also named accordingly.

For example. Ekahika jwara kashaya, dwahika jwara kashaya. Traahika jwara kashaya., sandhya jwara kashaya, nisajwara kashaya.

We find sarvadoshahara kashayas, 8 formulas are given suitable for all types of doshaja jwara. Likewise we find several formulas of jwarahara kashayas (fever curing decoctions) (2 formulas) mentioned for nisa jwara.

Rasoushadhas:

For vata pitta kapha jwara rasoushadhas namely Hiranyagarbha rasa with swarna, ganndhaka, manashila as important ingredients. Another is Sarabheswara rasa with parada, vatsanabha hingula haratala, gandhaka, as important ingredients.

We find many rasoushadhas mentioned which are equally effective to cure any kind of jwara (sarvajwara) such as Narayana rasa, vaishnavi rasa, lakshminarayana rasa, bhuteswara rasa, tripurantaka rasa, kalanadharasa, sambhavirasa, badrakali rasa etc. By observing the above nomenclature it appears that these formulations are named after diety whom he worshipped most. This type of attitude finding a formula which can be used to all types of fever resembles the thought process of present generation broad spectrum antibiotic. Exclusive rasoushadhas are prepared to treat targeting one individual disease. For example, Ekamurthy rasa for sita jwara, mahajwarankusa rasa for Ahika jwara, navanatharasa for ahika jwara and asthi gata jwara. We find 2 rasoushadha mentioned exclusively to be administered in high fever such as jwaradhumaketurasa, and pitamaha rasa. These rasoushadhas mainly contain parada, vatsanabha, hingula haratala and gandhaka.

Apart from this we observe several nasyas like manidruma nasya, hingu nasya, vyoshadi nasya etc., mentioned to cure exclusively for one individual jwara. Similarly different types of dhupa mentioned to treat different kinds of fevers like Ulukapaksha dhupa in chaturtika jwara, vacadi dhupa for vishama jwara. Author mentions food and activities to be undertaken during fever. Pathya and apathya mentioned for each type of jwara eg taruna jwara, vishama jwara etc. Author also mentions which are apathya applicable to all types of jwara.

The following are the rasoushadhas mentioned for the treatment of Jwara.

1) Hiranyagarbha rasam (swarna, tamra, rajita, pravala, gandhaka, manishila, talakam)

2) Sarabheswararasam (parada,, gandhaka, nabhi, hingulam).

3) Narasimharasam (parada, gandhakam, nabhi, nepalam)

4) Garudadhwajarasam (nabhi, rasam, abhrakam, gandhakam, hingulam)

6) Vaishnavirasa (hingulam, vatsanabhi)

7) Lakshminarayanaras (gandhakam, tuttham, tankanam, talakam)

8) Bhuteshwara rasam (paradam, visham, gandham, daradam)

9) Tripurantakarasam (rasam, gandham, abhrakam,)

10) Kalakandhara rasam (visham, manishila, sutam gandhakam, tankanam)

11) sanbhavirasam (parada, gandhaka, tankana, nepalam, gouripashanam)

12) Bhadrakalirasam (sutam, visham abhrakam, gandhakam, tankanam)

13) Bhuvaneshwararasam (gouriphashanam, abhrakam, vatsanabhi, manishila, rasam)

14) Umamaheshwara rasam (paradam, abhrakam)

15) Pitamaharasam (parad, nabhi, hingulam, loh andtamrabhasma, ayobhasma, talakam)

16) Bharatirasam (vacha, parada, gandham, abhrakam vatsanabhi)

17) Kalyanarasam (talakam, gandhaka, sankha ksharam)

18) Rasendrarasam (rasam, abhra, tamra, visham, gandhakam)

19) Viswambararasam (sutam, abhrakam, hingulam, visham,)

20) Ardhanareeswararasam (sutam, visham, vangam, hingulam)

21) Hutasana rasam (kushtam, gandham, visham,) .

22) Ekamurtirasam (musakapashanam),

23) DwimurtirasamNepalam, ulipashanam)

24) Chandabhanurasam (ksheeratuttham, talakam, shilakshara)

25) Suryapavakarasa (ullipashanam, goureepashanam, doddipashanam, maila tuttham, ksheera tuttham, nepalam, talakam)

26) Seetagajankusham (rasm, vatsanabhi, mailatuttham, karpari

27) Seetabhanjanarasam (maila&ksheeratuttham, ullipashan))

28) Panchamurtirasam (nepalam, ullipashanammailatuttham, ksheeratutham, talakam)

29) Mahajwarankusarasam (parade, visha, gandham, durtabeej)

30) Navanatharasam (nabhi, ulipashanam, mayuratuttham, palatuttham, rasam, doddipashanam, vasa, talakam, gandhakam)

31) Amoghastrarasam (vishatala, gouriphashanam, nabhi).

32) Chandrahasa rasam (paradam, gandhakam, daradam, tankanam, amrita, manishila)

33) Vishamrita rasam (nirvisham, rasam, gandham, nepalam, talakam)

34) Sadyajwarankusam (rasam, nagabhasma, vangabhasmam, nabhi)

35) Bhedhijwrankusa rasam (padarasam, hingulam, nabhi, gandham, tankanam,

36) Jwaradhumaketu rasam (padarasam gandham, hingulam, samudraphenam)

37) Navajwarebhankurasam (gandham, tankanam, rasam).

In jwara prakaranam about 37 new rasoushadhas are added. Many of these rasoushadhas we find parada, gandhaka, hingulam, gouree phashanam, ulipashanam, doddipashanam, talakam are the main ingredients and next preference is given to mailtuttham, ksheeratuttham, and tankanam.

Sannipata prakaranam :

The term Sannipata denotes a pathological vitiated condition of all three dosha.

In Vaidya chintamani author gives special importance to sannipata pakaranam and described in a separate chapter.

Sannipata jwara:

अतः परं प्रवक्ष्यामि सन्निपात ज्वर क्रमं । कंठे ललाटे हृदये स्वेदस्तंद्रा मतिभ्रमः ॥ १ ॥

अंगव्यथा शिरोरुक् च दाहस्सर्वांग नेत्रयोः । नेत्रे शोणित पीते च मूर्छा भ्रांतिः प्रलापकः ॥ २ ॥

हृच्छूलं गुंभनं हिक्का कास श्वासश्च हर्षणम् । सन्निपात ज्वरे घोरे वैद्यो विद्यात्तु लक्षणम् ॥३

Its important symptoms include sweating occurs over kantha (throat), lalata (fore head), tandra (drowsiness), matibhrama (giddiness in head) angapada, murcha (syncope), bhranti (hallucination, red and yellow colouration of the eye hridaya shula (angina pectoris), gumbhana (pulling pain of the heart), are the lakshana of the sannipata. These symptoms differ from the symptoms mentioned in Madhava nidanam and brihatrayee.

Sannipata types:

एकोल्बणास्त्रयस्तेस्युः द्विउलबणाश्च तथेति षट् । त्र्युल्बणश्च भवेदेको
विज्ञेयस्सतु सप्तमः ।। ४ ।। प्रवृद्ध मध्यहीनाश्च वातपित्त कफैश्च षट् ।
सन्निपात ज्वरस्यैवं स्युर्विशेषास्त्रयोदश ।। ५ ।।

Sannipata are of 13 types. They are, 3 varieties of sannipata with single dosha vitiation, 3 varieties of sannipata with two dosha vitiation, 6 varieties of sannipata with amsamsa kalpana of of dosa vitiation .

like this total sannipata are of 13 varities. They are

Vataja sannipata; pittaja sannipata; kaphaja sannipata;

vata pitta sannipata; vata sleshma sannipata; pitta kapha sannipata.

And the next classification sannipata as follows.

Hinavata madhyama pitta sleshmadhika sannipata. (acondition characterised by less of vata, middle state of pitta, excessive state of sleshma)

Hinavata, madhyama kapha, pittadhika sannipata

Hina pitta, madhyama kapha, vatadhikya sannipata.

Hinapitta, vata madhyama, sleshmadhikyata sannipata.

Hina kapha madhyama vata pittadhikya sannipata.

Hina kapha, madhyama pitta, vatadhikya sannipata lakshana.

Description of important varieties of sannipata :

Sandhikka sannipata:

स्वरूपं पूर्वमुच्छूलं शोफोवातिक वेदनाः ॥ २० ॥

कफस्तद्रातितापचसान् पाकि (sandhiika sanni pata)

Antaka sannipata; सदाहमोहस्तापश्च शिरःकंपः प्रलापनम् ॥ २२॥

वान्तिर्हिक्का ज्वरश्चैव ह्यन्तके सन्निपातके ।

hriddaha; प्रलाप ताप मोहाश्च कंठे वै वेदनाभ्रमः ॥ २५॥

विदाहोऽतितृषा कासो जाड्यं कंपः प्रलापनम् । स्वेदो ललाटे कंठेच रुग्दाहे सन्निपातके ॥ २६॥

Chittavibhrama sannipata: सर्वावयव वैकल्यं वातपित्त प्रकोपनम् । भ्रममोह भ्रुकुटिल गीतनृत्य प्रलापनम् ॥ २९ ॥ महाघोरस्सन्निपातो ज्ञातव्यश्चित्त विभ्रमः । (chitta vibhrama)

sitanga sannipata

सर्वांगं चंद्रवच्छीतं कास श्वास प्रकोपनम् ॥ ३१ ॥

हिक्का सर्वांग शैथिल्यं वान्ति सन्तापमूर्च्छनम् । अतिसारो गात्र कंपश्शीतांगे सन्निपातके ॥ ३२॥

Tandrika sannipata

बद्ध प्रलापस्तंद्राच जिह्वाश्यावा सकंटका । कठिना निर्द्रवा शुष्का सन्तापश्चातिसारकः ॥ ३४॥

श्वासः कंडूर्विरूपा दृक् तोयं स्रवति लोचनम् । ज्वरसत्त्वयुत्कटश्चैव तांद्रिके सन्निपातके ॥ ३५ ।

kanthakubja sannipata: अतिदाहशिशिरः कंप: कंधरस्यापि कुब्जता । विलापस्तापनं मूर्छा चांग शैथिल्यकंपनं ॥ ३७ छर्दिर्हिक्का गुंभनंच ह्युत्तमांग व्यथा तथा । सएवं सन्निपातोयं ज्ञातव्यः कंठकुब्जकः ॥ ३८

; karnika sannipata; bhugnanetra sannipata; raktoshta sannipata; pralapa sannipata; jihwaka sannipata; abhinyasa sannipata.

Above said all the thirteen varieties of sannipata though similar to the thirteen varieties sannipata mentioned by caraka in chikitsasthan but for them author has given special names worth noting. He considers sandhika, tandrika, pralapa, citta vibhrama, jihwaka, karnika sannipata are curable.

Author gives duration for each of the sannipata as follows

1 Sandhikka sannipata-7 days

2 Antaka sannipata-10 days

3 Hriddaha sannipata-20 days

4 chittavibhrama sannipata 21 days

5 sitanga sannipata 15 days

6 tandrika sannipata 25/7 days

7 kanthakubja sannipata 13 days

8 karnika sannipata 3 months

9 bhugnanetra sannipata 8 days

10 raktoshta sannipata 10 days

11 pralapa sannipata 14 days

12-jihwaka sannipata 16 days

13 abhinyasa sannipata.15 days

Patient may get death after the occurrence of sannipata jwara on 2nd, 3rd 5th, 7th .10th, 12th, and 21st day.If the patient crosses these stipulated days survives.

Patient may get death or he may get relieved from sannipata after the occurrence of sannipataja jwara on 7th, 9th, 11th 14th, 18th 22nd day .In the case of pitta prakopa after 10 days, in the case of kapha prakopa after 12 days, in the case of vata prakopa after after 7 days the patient will get death. Durinng this period dosa, dhatu mala paka will take place, which leads to death or relief from the sannipata . The above concept appears to be novel.

Dosa, dhatu and mala paka:

Author mentions that dosa, dhatu and mala paka should be observed by the following symptoms.

निद्रानाशो ह्रदिस्तम्भो विष्टंभो गौरवाऽरुची ॥ ६४ ॥

अरतिर्बलहानिश्च धातुनां पाक लक्षणं

This particular stanzas taken from bhavaprakasha.

Author mentioning of dhatupaka lakshana states that nidranasa (insomnia), hrdayastmbha (constriction sensation of heart), malabaddhata, gaurava (heaviness), aruchi (loss of taste), vyakulata, balahani (loss of strength) are the lakshanas of dhatupaka .

Notes: *Dhatu Paka (suppuration or destruction) is a pathological and unfavorable condition for body. It is a condition in which tissues are severely destructed in quick time. This leads to manifestation of many diseases and loss of immunity and strength.*

Dosapaka lakshana:

दोषप्रकृतिगावित्वं लघुता ज्वर देहयोः ।। ६५ ।।

इंद्रियाणांच वैमल्यं दोषाणां पाक लक्षणं

Normalisation of dosa, laghuta, and indiya nirmalata are the alkshanas.

Sannipata jwara kashayas:

Kashayas are formulated to cure sannipata jwara. These kashayas are prepared in order to be administered exclusively in a particular type of sannipata and named after that particular sannipata itself.

Eg.. Sandhika sannipata kashayam, atanka sannipata kashayam etc.Likewise every sannipata is treated with kashaya which is specifically prepared for it.

Important ingredients of these kashayas include the following drugs.maha bala, pippalimulam, chitramulam chavya, trkatu sarpakshi, varuna panchakola, kasmari, bilva etc.

Apart from this, author specifies two kashayams considers to treat all types of sannipata, and one of them named as dasamula kashayam. Important ingredients include dasamula, pippali, jayanti, bhunimba and vacha. Similarly Rasoushadhas are also prepared exclusively treat individual type of sannipata eg., Vijaya bhirava rasa prepared for Atanka sannipata.

Rasoushadhas for sannipata:

Important rasoushadhas mentioned for sannipata are Sringara bhirava rasa for the treatment of hriddaha sannipata, madana bhirava rasa for the treatment chitta vibhrama sannipata, Ananda bhairavarasa for sitanga sannipata. Mano bhairava rasa in Tanbdrika sannipata etc.

The important ingredients of these rasoushadhas include Suddha parada (processed mercury), suddha manshila (processed realgar) suddha gandhaka (sulphur (suddha tankana (processed borax) tamra, (copper bhasma), vanga (tin) and triphala .

The diet mainly recommended are dadhi (curd), butter milk (takra) and rice, narikela jala and ksheranna and madhu.

The following are the different types of Anjana mentioned by the author for sannipata.

Anjana:

Notes: *Anjana is a paste applied to the inner part of eyelids.*

The following are the new formulation about anjana. They are kanadyanjana, rasnadyanjana, turangalaladyanjana, sireesha beejadyanjana, prabhodhadya njana, bala suryodaya njana, bhairavanjanam, vijnanajanam, veerabhadradyanjanam, prakasanjanam, and divyanjanam. Author is of the view that all these anjanas are capable of curing all types sannipata .In these anjana we find following important ingredients such as Pippali, maricham, karanja, vasa, triphala, trikatu, manishila, rasna, sireesha beejam, turanga lala (saliva of horse) haridra, brihati phala, vakula beejam, eranda beejam, hingu.

In the preparation for most of these anjana he advocates mardana with gomutra, basta mutra, madhu and is applied to the eyes.

Dhupa for Sannipata: Even while describing dhupa too we find that particular type of dhupa indicated in particular type of sannipata. Eg.Nirgundi dhupam indicated in sandhika sannipata .Nagarjuna dhupa, kshetrapala dhupa indicated in all types of sannipata.These are the new formulations by the author and includes the following ingredients like nirgundi, sarsapa, nimba, agaru, karpura. And also, sarpakurpasam, khara vistam, saranga vista, kola vista, sikhipaksha, vrischika, bringa paksha form part of dhupa dravya.

Nasyam for Sannipata:

Similarly we find separate nasyam are exclusively prepared for some of the important sannipata. Nasyam prepared from kumbhodbhava etc drugs in the treatment of chitta vibhrama sannipata. Nasyam prepared from pippali manishila, talakam etc indicated in tandrika sannipata. Apamarga, trikatu, katu tumbee etc indicated in kanta kubja sannipata. Nasyam prepared from maricha, kana, and lavana, indicated in karnika sannipata. Nasyam prepared from maricham, aswagandha etc indicated in bhugna netra sannipata. Nasyam prepared from durvarasam dadima pushpa rasam indicated in raktasteevi sannipata. Bhasmeswara nasyam with important ingredients like nabhi, maricha, bhasma etc indicated in all types of sannipata. Arkeshwara nasyam with the important ingredients like bhasma added with maricha churna indicated in all types of sannipata.

In treatment of sannipata metals like suvarnarajita, mukta, pravala, rudraksha added with yastimadhukam, putrajeevi etc drugs macerated in sthanya and applied, and this is indicated in all types of sannipata and also in all diseases.

Like wise we find kulattha, katphala prepared in to lepa and applied on karna mula sopha.

Rasoushadhas mentioned sannipata:

we observe the following rasoushadhas are the new formulations mentioned by the author .The main ingredients given in brackets.

1) Bhuta bhairava rasam (rasam, gandhaka, tamrabhasma)
2) Vijayabhairavarasam (rasam, nabhi, vangabhasma, nagabhasma, abhraka bhasma,)

3) .Sangarabhairavarasam (tamra bhasma, lohabhasma, triksharam, parada)

4) Madana bhairavarasam (rasam gandhakam, manishila, saindhavalavanam, tamram)

5) Anandabhairavarasam (tankanam, hingulam, gandham, haraveeryam talakam, teekshnam, vangam, tamram, nagam) .

6) Manobhairava rasam ((triksharam, panchalavanam, tamram, rasam)

7) swancchanda bhairavarasam (rasam, gandham, tankanam, visham, vangabhasma)

8) Kalyanabhairavarasam (rasam visham, visham (snake poison), gandhakam, nagam, vangam)

9) Vidarana bhairavarasam (rasam, tamrabhasma, vangabhasma)

10) Sannipata bhairava rasa (sutam, visham, abhraka, gandhaka, nagam, tankanam) .

11) Karunyabhairavarasam (rasam, abhraka bhasma,

12) Siddhabhairava rasa (paradam, talakam)

13) Karavala bhairavarasa (haraveeryam, ramatham, triksharam, gandhakam, panchalavanam, nabhi)

Many of the rasoushadhas prepared in such a way that they could cure one particular sannipata.

Rasoushadhas effective againist all sannipata:

Author mentions the following rasoushadas, which are equally effective againist all the sannipata. For example,

1) Veeravikramaras (paradam, tankana, gandhakam, vishatindukabeeja, saindhavalavana)

2) Trivikramarasam (sutam, visham, talakam)

3) Jayavikramarasa (visham, manishila, talakam, gandhakam, tankanam) .

4) Mahendrarasam (Garalam, rasam, talakam, manishila, doddipashanam)

5) lokeshwara rasam (talakam, daradam, rasam, nabhi,)

6) Mahabhairavarasam (rasabhasma, tamrabhasma, lohabhasma, abhrakabhasma, kantabhasma)

7) Mrityunjayarasam (abhrakam, talakam, haraveeryam, gandhakam, samudraphenam)

8) Pranayanalarasam (rasam, nabhi, hingulam, tankanam, triksharam, panchalavanam)

9) Pasupatasra rasam (ullipashanam, goureepashanam dwituttham, nepalam, talakam, nabhi)

10) Rogavidavaranarasam (haraveerya, vatsanabhi, tankana,, makshikam talakam, gandhakam, abhrakam, tripashana)

11) Rajarajeshwararasam (haraveeryam, gandhakam, talakam, makshikam, trikshara)

12) Kalagnirudrarasam (trikshara, panchalavana, rasam, nabhi)

13) Mritasanjeevirasam (Sutam, visham, gandham, hingulam, katukarohini)

14) Dhnvantarirasam (rasam, nabhi, swarnabhasma, lohabhasma, mutyabhasma, triksharam, vangabhasma)

15) Phanibhushanarasam (talaka, daradam, vanga, naga, abhrak)

16) Sannipatadavanalarasam (talakam, nagam, vangam, haraveeryam, tankanam, trikshara, panchalavana, goureepashanam, nabhi)

17) Rogabhanjanarasam (rasam, abhrakam, tamram, nabhi)

18) Kalabhairavarasam (talakam, gandhakam, tamram, haraveeryam, tankanam, triksharam, saindhavalavanam, bolam maricham)

19) Pranagnikumararasa (rasam, visham, abhrakaka, gandham)

20) Sudivyagnikumararasam (haraveeryam, visham)

21) Uttamagnirasa (rasam, abhraka, kanta, loha)

22) Viswambararasam (rasam abhrakam, hingulam, visha, talakam)

23) Mahakalagnirudrarasam (hingulam, talakam, sutam, manishila,, tankanam, gandhakam)

24) Yoganadharasam (rasam, gandhakam, tuttham, manishila, hemamakshikam, garalam, hingulam, loham, tamra).

25) Vishama suchikarasam (sutam, sarpavisham, nabhi,

26) Sannipata kulantakarasam (rasam, gandhakam, nabhi trikatuka)

27) Panchavaktra rasam (sutam, visham, gandham, maricham, tankanam, kana)

28) Parasuramakutharam (nagabhasma, gandhakam, rasam, tankanam, nabhi)

All the above 28 yogas mentioned to cure all the varities of sannipata. Thus author has advised two separate sets of rasoushadhas one to treat individual varieties of sannipata, and the other is to treat all varieties of sannipata.

Sarvajvara Santi measures:

Author mentions the following measures for sarva jvara santi as follows

ज्वरे रुद्रजपं कुर्यान्महारुद्रं महाज्वरे । महारुद्रं जपेद् रौद्रे वैष्णवे तद्द्वयं जपेत् ॥४॥To relieve from samanya jwara a person has to read rudrajapa. In case of mahajvara he has to chant maharudrajapa.In case of vaishnava jvara he has to read two maharudrajapa.

Aṣṭa Jvara Santi

वेदानां श्रवणं हितस्य चरण विप्रस्य संतर्पणम् ॥९॥

कृष्णस्य स्मरण शुभस्य करणं द्रव्यस्य विश्राणनम् । अश्वत्थभ्रमण सुरत्नधरणं दीनस्य संरक्षणम्॥१०॥ हन्यादष्टविधं ज्वरं कुमुदिनीनाथो यथोग्रं तमः । सहस्रनेत्रस्य सहस्रबाहो सहस्रवक्त्रस्य सहस्रमूर्धः । सहस्रपादस्य सहस्रनामः

सहस्त्रनाम्नां पठनं ज्वरघ्नम् ॥ ११ ॥ गणेश्वरं वा गरुडेश्वरं वा गौरीश्वरं वा दिवसेश्वरं वा महेश्वरीं वा कुलदैवतं वा संपूजयेत्तज्ज्वरिणांप्रशस्तम् ॥ १२ ॥

The following measures relieve one from astajwara santi as follows, listening to veda, good behavior, donating food to bramhana, praying lord Krishna, pradakshina to aswatha vriksha wearing suitable gems stones in rings and helping poor people.

Kshaya prakaranam: Author gives much importance to the disease kshaya and describes it vividly.

Kshaya is a pathological state in which there is decrease in quality, quantity and or functioning of the elements (dhatus) of the body. But in this context author considers it as a disease by itself analogus to rajayakshma.

Lakshanas of Kshaya prakarana mentioned in Vaidyachintamani are mostly derived from madhavanidana. Depending on the necessity author has taken leverage in removing certain slokas and also added of his own at some palces.

In this we find peculiar reference about members of kshaya.

Members of Ksaya:

क्षयरोगे ज्वरो राजा तस्य पत्नी तु कामिला । चमूपतिः पांडुरोगो रक्तपित्तस्तु पुत्रकः ॥१॥ सौख्यं शोभतिसारौच मंत्रिणौ श्वासकासकौ । गुठचारौ वातिपित्तौ वाजिनौ वान्तिकारुची ॥ २ ॥ ग्रहण्यशों गुल्म शूला गायकास्तूर्य वाद्यकाः । शिरोमणिशिरोरोगः पीनसश्चात् पत्रकम् ॥ ३॥ भक्तव्देषो भद्रपीठं भद्रदन्ती च साहसः । स्वर क्षयस्तु तांबूलं सत्वहानिश्चत् चंदनं ॥४॥ बलक्षयो भुजबलं निष्ठ्यूतिर्हिमवालुकः । अनेक रोगानुगतो बहुरोग पुरोगमः ॥५॥ एतेन परिवारेण रोगराजो विराजते । असाध्योऽयं महारोगो सहस्त्रदिवसावधिः ॥६॥

In kshaya prakaranam we find peculiar description about the members of kshaya as follows. In the kingdom of ksaya roga jwara is the king, kamala is his wife, panduroga is general of army, raktapittam is the son etc, sopha and atisara are pleasure, swasa and kasa are ministers. Vatapitta are spies.vanti and aruchi are horses. Grahani, sula, arsa, gulma and sula are singers and orchestra etc.

In the family of ksaya, many diseases will stand in the front like members of kingdom. Kshaya considered as raja of all diseases. Hence it is also called as Rajayakshma. It is an incurable disease as it is very difficult to cure. Limitation of this dsease is thousand days. Like other diseases karmavipaka and jyotissabhipraya described for this disease, (earlier described).

Nidana (causative factors) :

Rajayakshma occurs because of four reasons viz.:

1) Vagavarodha (suppression of the urges ie urine, faeces, sneezing etc.).

2) Dhatu kshaya (depletion of tissues).

3) Sahasa (doing activities beyond his capacity).

4) Vishamabhojana (irregular regimen of food).

It is of 2 types

Anuloma kshaya and Viloma kshaya

Anuloma kshaya occurs because of obstruction in the srotas by vitiated kapha etc dosa.

Pratiloma kshaya occurs because of sukra dhatu kshinata leading to ksinata of other dhatus. Just like moon reduces subsequently from purnima to amavasya, similarly because of yakshma roga, the patient slowly gets ksinata.

kshya lakshanas

Mentioning of the main characteristics of kshaya author mentions that tapa (temperature) in shoulders, head and lateral parts of the body, burning sensation in the hands and legs .Fever in all parts of the body are the important characteristics of kshaya.

Eleven, six and three lakshana of kshaya:

Just as Brihatrayee author also mentions about syndromes or group of symptoms unique for kshaya ie ekadasa (eleven), shadrupa (six) and trividharupa (group of three symptoms)

Ekadasa rupa kshaya : The following are the eleven symptoms of Kshaya.They are peswarabhedha, vatajasula, skanda-parsva sankocha (bending of the shoulders and lateral side of the body), jwara, daha, atisara, vamana, sirobhara (heaviness of the head), annadwesha (dislike for food), kasa and kannthdwamsa (bending of the neck) .

Shadrupa kshaya: kasa, atisara, parsvapida, swarabheda aruchi, jwara are Six types of kshaya lakshanas

Trividha kshaya: jwra, kasa, rakta roga (disease of blood)

are the three tpes of characters of kshaya .

Incurability of Kshaya:

Author describing the incurability of kshaya mentions that

Whitish discolouration of eyes Strong dislike for food urdhwaswasa (prolonged expirational dyspnea) prameha (increased frequency of urine and turbidity) persons are incurable.

Author gives description that in kshata kshaya urosula (pain in the chest), rakta vamana (vomiting in the blood) excessive cough, rakta varna in mutra, pain and stiffness of feet are the symptoms of incurability in kshata kshaya.

"Param dina sahasram tu yadi Jeevati manavaha subhishgbhirupakrantu starunassosha peeditah" means if the patient lives for one thousand days then he can be treated.

Vimasati kshaya:

Author of Vaidyachintamani elaborately describes vimsati kshaya.

The following are vimsati Kshaya.

कारयेत्कदलीं दिव्यां पत्रैस्सर्वत्र संयुताम् ॥७॥ फलपूगेन संयुक्तां सुवर्णस्य पलेन तु । यथा विभवतः कुर्याद्वस्त्रेणावेष्ट्य सूत्रकैः ॥८॥
ब्राह्मणान्भोजयेच्चापि भक्ष्यैर्नानाविधैश्शुभैः । होमंच कारयेत्तत्र यथावताणेन च ॥ ९ ॥ तस्मै तां कदलीं दद्यात् वस्त्रालंकार पूर्विकाम् । पजिताय दरिद्राय व्रतस्थायात्म वेदिने ॥ १० ॥ धर्मज्ञायातिदान्ताय मंत्रेणानेन तां क्षयी ।
हिरण्यगर्भ पुरुष परात्पर जगन्मय ॥ ११॥ रंभादानेन देवेश क्षयं क्षपय मे प्रभो । पुण्याहवाचनं कार्यं ब्राह्मणैर्वेदपारगै ॥ १२ ॥ शिष्टैरिष्टैर्बंधुभिश्च सहभोजनमाचरेत् ।s

धर्मशास्त्रण्यविज्ञाय प्रायश्चित्तं दधाति यः ॥ १३ ॥

राजयक्ष्मा भवेत्तस्य रोगपीडातिदारुणा । पर्वोक्तेन विधानेन प्रदद्यात्प्रतिरूपकम् ॥१४॥ क्षयरोगस्य घोरस्य वक्ष्यमाणकृतिस्वयं । राजयक्ष्माकृशतनुश्शरचाप धनुस्तथा ॥ १५ ॥ दक्षिणेन करेणापि सभयंकृततर्जनः । दधत्रिनेत्रं दंष्ट्राभ्यां दष्टोष्ठो हन्तुमुद्यतः ॥ १६ ॥

Origin of Ksaya:

Here Author narrates story related to origin of kshaya that goddess parvati after praying Shankara asks him to say about 20 varieties of kshaya. Then god shankara replies and says that the people who are vice and commit the killing of revered woman like king's wife or wife of acharya etc., develops the disease. The sequence of the development of the disease is as follows:

The person when kills woman of reverence then the sin accrues in him but only after some time, it leaves the sthula deha and gets yatana deha then enters into mutkana kupa (hollow pit) which is highly offensive, disgusting and spread with full of criminals. These criminal people take birth after mourning for hundred long years as per pitrumana and after lapse of some period suffer from Kshaya. And in the beginning of the disease he suffers from fever, pandu, sotha, kamila, grahani etc and all these diseases many a time run a chronic course makes the patient extremely weak and emaciated.

Another important contribution by him is stating about the concept of what type of kshaya occurs at what age is amazing. It is shown in table form.

Kshaya Roga According to Number of Birth

प्रथमः पंचमे वर्षे व्दितीयस्सप्तमे समे । तृतीयश्चाष्टमेब्दे तु चतुर्थः दशमेऽब्दिके ॥ ९२॥ पंचमो व्दादशे वर्षे षष्ठश्चापि त्रयोदशे । सप्तम क्षय सम्प्राप्तिर्वत्सरे च चतुर्दशे ॥ ९३ ॥ अष्टमष्षोडशे वर्षे नवमस्तु तदुत्तरे । दशम नवमस्तु तदुत्तरे । दशम क्षय सम्प्राप्तिर्वत्सरेष्टादशे तथा । । ९४॥ एकादशः क्षयश्चापि तथा विंशति वत्सरे । व्दादशः पंचविंशेच त्रयोदश उदीरितः ॥ ९५ ॥ त्रिंशें वयसि संप्राप्ते महादुःखकरस्सदा । चतुर्दश क्षय पराप्तिः पंचत्रिंशेच वत्सरे ॥ ९६॥

क्षयः पंचदशश्चापि सप्तत्रिंशेच वत्सरे । षोडष क्षय सम्प्राप्तिरष्टत्रिंशेच वत्सरे ॥ ९७ ॥ क्षयस्सप्तदशश्चैव चत्वारिंशेच वत्सरे । अष्टादशः क्षयश्चैव त्रिचत्वारिंशवत्सरेः ॥ ९८ ॥ पंचचत्वारिंशके च क्षयस्त्वेकोनविंशति; । अष्टचत्वारिंशके च विंशति क्षयसंभवः ॥ ९९ ॥ ईदृग्विधो महादेवि प्रतिजन्मच पीडयेत् । जन्मनि प्रथमे देवि रक्तक्षय उदाहृतः ॥ १०० ॥ व्दितीये राजयक्ष्माच संतापस्तु तृतीयके । चतुर्थे जन्मनि प्राप्ते मूर्छा क्षय उदाहृतः ॥ १०१ ॥ पंचमे शोष संज्ञश्च षष्ठेच वमन क्षयः । सप्तमे ग्रहणी शूलमष्टमे शोफनामकः ॥ १०२ ॥ नवमे शुष्कनामाच दशमे चातिसारकः । एकादशेच मंदाग्निः व्दादशेच विवर्णकः ॥ १०३ ॥ त्रयोदशे जन्मनि च ह्वजीर्ण क्षय संभवः ।

चतुर्दशेतित्कनामा ह्युद्गारस्तु तदुत्तरे ॥ १०४ ॥ षोडषे जन्मनि प्राप्ते दाहक्षय समुद्भवः । भवे सप्तदशे चैव तंद्रा क्षय उदाहृतः ॥ १०५ ॥ जन्मन्यष्टादशे चैव हिध्माक्षय समुद्भवः । जन्मन्येकोनविंशेच दारुण क्षय संभवः ॥ १०६ ॥ ॥ विंशे जन्मनि संप्राप्ते हरिद्राक्षय सम्भवः । स्त्रीहतया पाप संभूतो विविधं गुणमाश्रितः ॥ १०७ ॥

Table showing what type of kshaya occurring at what age and which birth.

In What birth	At what age	Type of Kshaya
In the 1st birth	5 years	Rakta Kshaya
In the 2nd birth	7 years	Raja yakshma
In the 3rd birth	8 years	SantapaKshaya
In the 4th birth	10 years	Murcha Kshaya
In the 5th birth	12 years	Sosha Kshaya
In the 6th birth	13 years	Vamana Kshaya
In the 7th birth	14 years	Grahanee shula Kshaya
In the 8th birth	16 years	Sopha Kshaya
In the 9th birth	17 years	Susha Kshaya
In the 10th birth	18 years	Atisara Kshaya
In the 11th birth	20 years	Mandagni Kshaya

In the 12th birth	25 years	Vivarna Kshaya
In the 13th birth	30 years	Ajeerna Kshaya
In the 14th birth	35 years	Tikta Kshaya
In the 15th birth	38 years	Udgara Kshaya
In the 16th birth	38 years	Daha Kshaya
In the 17th birth	40 years	Tandra Kshaya
In the 18th birth	43 years	Hikka Kshaya
In the 19th birth	45 years	DarunaKshaya
In the 20th birth	48 years	Haridra Kshaya@

We get another set of symptoms termed as gunas (etc gunascha Vijneyaha Kshayarogeshu Sooribhihi) of kshayarogas. But these gunas are more or less similar to the symptoms mentioned in ekadasarupa (eleven symptoms of kshaya), shadrupa (six symptoms of kshaya) mentioned for Rajayakshma.

Notes:

Kshaya a disease mentioned in Vaidyacintamani is a new name given to Rajayakshma referred to in Ayurveda texts. Rajayakshma is a syndrome consisting of diseases associated with wasting (kshaya) of various tissues including rasa and ojas causing immunodeficiency resulting in opportunistic infections like tuberculosis. Kshaya (tissue depletion) may also be the result of cancers comparable to cachexia. The term rajayakshma has been also used interchangeably with tuberculosis.

Important characteristic feature of Vimsati Kshaya are as follows

Rakta Kshaya: On every eighth day or tenth day, or for fifteen days, or for one month, bimonthly or six monthly person will have bleeding from nose, mouth, rectum, or ears occur and suffers from weakness, loss of appetite, cough with expectoration. Sweda, sarvanga santapa, nissatwa (weakness), murcha, excessive cachexia, kantihinata (loss of glow), mandagni, malabaddhata (constipation), kasa and kapha are the lakshanas.

Though rajayakshma mentioned as equal disease to kshaya but Author includes Rajaykshma as one of the categories of kshaya and also mentions separate causative factors for it.

The other kshayas mentioned by the author are Santapa kshaya, Murcha kshaya, Sosha kshaya, Vamana kshaya, Grahanee shula kshaya, Sopha kshaya, Sushka kshaya, atisara kshaya, mandagni kshaya, pandu kshaya, Ajeerna kshaya, tikta kshaya, udgara kshaya, kasa kshaya, daha kshaya, swara kshaya, hidhma kshaya and haridra kshaya.

All these kshaya possess almost similar symptoms, but naming of each kshaya separately probably based on severety of a particular symptom. Eg. The naming of Haridra kshaya probably based on the symptom of yellowish discolouration of all parts of the body. Above mentioned different types of kshaya simulates cachexia resulted due to malignant condition of individual organs. According to author all these Kshaya result from the sin of killing of woman. But in some kshaya he mentions it due to the sin of previous birth. But it is amazing to note mentioning of survival period to these kshayas separately. This resembles indicating life span for different cancers seen present day.

The following is the survival period showing against the name of the each of the Kshaya

Name of the Kshaya survival Period

1) Rakta Kshaya	Suffers 5 months
2) Rajaya Kshaya	6 months survival
3) Santapa Kshaya	Suffers 9 months, later he will live or die
4) Murcha Kshaya	Suffers for 7 months, later lives or will die
5) Sosha Kshaya	Survives only for 8 months
6) Vamana Kshaya	Survives only for 1 year
7) Grahanee Shula Kshaya	Suffers for 2 years later death ensues
8) Sopha Kshaya	Suffers for 5 years
9) Sushka Kshaya	Suffers for 7 years
10) Atisara Kshaya	Suffers for 2 years
11) Mandagni Kshaya	Suffers for 10 years
12) Pandu Kshaya	Suffers for 9 years
13) Shula Kshaya	
14) Tikta Kshaya	Suffers for 12 years
15) Kasa Kshaya	Suffers for 8 years
16) Daha Kshaya	Suffers for 8 years
17) Tandra Kshaya	Suffers for 10 years
18) Hidma Kshaya	Suffers for 10 years
19) Daruna Kshaya	
20) Haridra Kshaya	Survives for 8 months.

Thus stipulating time period for each of the Kshaya denotes that they were in a position to identify the given clinical condition accurately inspite of having several similar symptoms present in each of the kshaya. It can be presumed that they used to record the period of suffering for each clinical condition out of academic interest. We observe that while mentioning symptoms and causative factors of a disease he also advocates medicines simultaneously appears unconventional. It is interesting to note that author version stating that the patient after specified period of suffering will live for 100 years. Eg. Shula Kshaya.

Important rasoushadhas mentioned for ksaya are as follows:

Mahakanaka sundara rasa; Nilakantha rasa; Trailokya cintamani rasa

Rajamriganka rasa; Suvarna bhupathi rasa; Hemabhraka rasa sindhura

Mrigankarasa; Pancamrita rasa; Vasanta kusumakararasa; Sankeswararasa

Hara rudra rasa; Sankha garbha pottali rasa; Hemagarbharasa; Kumudeswara rasa; Svayamagni kumara rasa; Navaratna raja mriganka rasa; Purna chandrodaya rasa; Pippalyadi rasayana; Hastikarni rasa; Hemagarbha pottali rasa; Kantavallabharasa; Lokanatharasa; Aswagandha rasayana; Talaka sinndhura; Varaladi lehya; ksudra harikai lehya; babbuladi lehya; avsadi lehya; kushmanda ghrta; Pancasara ghrta; Aswagandhadi ghrtaPippalyadi ghrta; Pippalyasava; Drakshasava Kharjurasava; Surya prabhagutika; Laghu siva gutika; Drakshadi churna;

Eladi churna; Aswagandha churna; Trikatvadi churna; Jatiphaladi churnam

Aswgandha bala akshadi tailam; Chandanadi tailam; Ksira tailam.

The above rasoushadhi having the following main ingredients such as parada. Gandhaka, abhraka, kantabhsma, loha, guggulu vaikrata hasma, rajata, mashila, tankana, trikatu, vatsanabha pippali and aswagandha.

All these ingredients incidentally are rasayana and capable of tackling the depleted condition of rasadhatu. (ksaya). Hara rudra rasa considered uttama among all the rasaushadhi. Chandanadi tailam, aswagandha bala lakshadi tailam proven oils for the use of massage. For nourishment aja dugdha and godudha are liberally used, these rasoshadhas are generally given in the dose of gunja or 125 mg a day.

Exclusive formula to improve rasadhatu:

Kwatha is preparation with guduchi, ardraka yava or milk boiled with marica is to be taken in night to increase rasadhatu and also it is useful in the treatment of pthisis.

Amavata and rheumatism:

Author says that improperly formed rasadhatu results in ama and cause Amavata.

Clinical features of amavata are akin to Rheumatism on modern parlance. The clinical features include are pains all over the body, loss of taste, thirst, lack of enthusiasm, heaviness, fever, indigestion and swelling of the body parts. Just as any other disease author gives karma vipaka and jyotissastrabhipraya for this disease also (described earlier)

It depicts that poor digestive capacity causes improper digestion of food resulting in the formation of ama (improperly digested food) this ama associated with vata moves quickly to the seats of kapha and coats dhamani with waxy material, hence produces weakness and heaviness of the heart which becomes the seat of the disease. It also affects simultaneously the joints of the body produces stiffness of the body and also becomes a cause for many other diseases. It becomes incurable when it affects all joints of hands feet, feet, head, heels, waist knee and thigh etc., causing painful swelling which shifts from joint to joint since dosas move place to other. The pain will be severe and resembles that of a scorpion sting. If it associates with pitta causes burning sensation and redness of the of the affected part, if vata is predominant pain will be severe and if kapha is predominant loss of movement and itching will be seen. It is considered incurable if all dosas are involved

The formmulations for amavata are described in vaidyacintamani as follows.

Rasnadi kashaya, maha rasnadi kashaya, laghurasnadi kashaya, rasna dwadasa kashaya sunthyadi kashaya sathyadi kshaya, dasamuladi kashaya, ajamodadi chrna

Panca sama churna, triphaladi churna, punarnavadi churna, vaiswanara churna chitrakadi churna, amavatari rasa, vatari rasa, udaya bhaskara rasa abhayadi gutika, erandai gutika, hari gutika simhanda guggulu, haritaki guggulu, yogaraja guggulu brihat saindhavadya taila, methipaka soubhagya sunthi paka satapushpadi lepa .

Important ingredients used in these formulations considered effective againist amavata are guggulu, erandamula, rasna, ativisa, devadaru, vacaharitakki pippali, marica, trivritpunarnava citraka guduchi, vatsanabha.

And also, parada, gandhaka, tamra, suddha tutha given much preference.

Pathya (benbeficial diet) : In Amavata Ruksha sweda (sweating procedure without applying oil), langhana, vata and kapha hara ahara, shunti, eranda and patola are considered beneficial. In short all dipana padartha (appetizers) are considered as pathya.

Apathya: Apathya in Amavata are curd, fish, jaggery, milk, polluted water heavy food are contra indicated.

SOPHA: The term Shotha or sopha refers to swelling or inflammation. It is also known as Svayathu in ayurveda. It is a wide term covering local swellings to inflammation of internal organs such as bronchitis, pancreatitis etc.

Explaining pathogenesis of sopha author mentions that vitiated vata, vitiated raktapitta, vitiated kapha reaches sira (vessels) ultimately causing srotavarodha (obstruction in the channels) . This srotovarodha produces stagnation of vitiated dosha in twacha and mamsa (skin and muscle) and develops sopha (swelling) . Author mentions sopha is of 9 types.

Vataja, pittaja, kaphaja, vatapittaja, vatakphaja, pitta kaphaja, sannipataja, abhighataja and visaja. Mentioning the causative factors for sopha he states if the person suffering from krsa (emaciation), balaksaya (loss of strength) takes diet containg ksara, amla, tiksna, ruksa, guru (aalkaline, sour, pungent, dry and heavy) ahara (food), and also habit of taking mrd bahkshana (earth eating), incompletely cooked food, polluted food, incompatible food (viruddha ahara) .

Author did not describe sannipataja sopha but adds up dwandwaja sopha (resulted beacause of 2 doshas) .

In abhighataja sopha (swelling resulted due to injury etc), apart from abhighta with weapons knife etc., we find mention of contact of bhallataka, kapikachu etc also mentioned as causative factors of sopha.

Under vishaja sopha contact of urine and faeces of poisionous animals and plants, poisonous gases, garavisa (slow and accumulated poisions) sopha gets developed. This type of sopha will be mridu cancala and spreading in nature. He mentions that dosha pertaining to amasaya produces urdhwa bhaga shotha (oedema of upper part of the body) and dosha from malashaya produces adho bhag shotha (oedema of lower part of the body).

Astavidha sopha:

Krtrima visa sopha:

कृत्रिमं विषमाश्रित्य पूर्णं शोफ समुद्भवः । दारुणश्शर्मगात्रेषु ज्वरो रोम्णां च जृंभणम् ॥ २१ ॥ भारश्च सर्वगात्राणां वैवर्ण्यं नेत्रयुग्मके । मलबंधश्शातिसार आध्मानं चाग्निमांद्यकम् ॥ २२ ॥ अन्नद्वेषो ह्याजीर्णत्वं श्वासपूर्वा च वेदना । हिक्का हिध्मा च हृत्तापः शिरोभ्रमणकंपनम् ॥ २३ ॥ वैरूप्यं चांगवैकल्यं वैवश्य क्रोधसंभवः । राजपत्नी राजपुत्री स्वपुत्रीणां वधेन च ॥ २४ ॥ पापेन कृत्रिमः शोफ उद्भवेत्पीडयेत् सदा । द्विकालं चतुरो मासान् संपूर्णं सेवयेन्नरः ॥ २५ ॥ वर्षाभू लेह्यकं चैव ह्यामामाहेश्वरं 1 रसम् । गंधर्वरसविख्यातं मंडूरादिरसायनम् ॥ २६॥

कौशिकस्य च तैलस्य लेपः कृत्रिमशोफनुत् ।

Severe oedema will be produced because of kritrima visa in skin and in all parts of the body. Vivarnata (discoloration) in netra, malabaddhata (constipation), atisara (diarrhoea), annadwesha, urdhwa swasa, hikka, hidma, hridaya santapa (rise of te temperature in heart) angavaikalya (temporary deformity in body parts krodha (anger) are the characteristics of sopha produced by kritrima visa.

Mentioning the karmavipaka of the disease shotha that it is produced because of killing of rajapatni, rajaputri and his own daughter. Punarnavalehya administered 2 times a day for 4 months.

Other rasoushadhas used are Umamaheswararasa, gandharva rasa and manduradi rasayana. Kaushika taila indicated for external massage. This taila is commonly prescribed by him as an external application.

Pashana dosha sopha:

आखुपाषाणगौयौं च कर्परी बर्हिणी शिला ॥ २७ ॥

मूलिकामिलितं वाथ सेवयेदेकमेव चेत् । पाषाणदोषो मासौ द्वौ हृन्मध्यं च समाश्रितः ॥ २८ ॥ आम्लं तक्रं च लवणं दधिभक्तं दिने दिने । दाडिमी बीजपूरश्च चिंचाम्लं चूतमाम्लकम् ॥ २९ ॥ जंबुजंबीरजाम्लं च भुक्तवंतं तु मानुषम् । एषां निमित्तमात्राच्च पुराकृतमहैनसः ॥ ३० ॥ दारुणः शोफ आविः स्याच्छिरोभ्रमणकंपने । हिक्का हिध्मा तथोद्गारो ज्वरः शीतं शिरोव्यथा ॥

(pashana dosha lakshana)

Akupashana, gauripashana (arsenic oxide) shilajith (mineral pitch) nila tutha (blue vitriol) if administered Without doing sodhana or without medicinal plant that will affect heart within 2 months and during this period if one consumes amlam, takram and lavanam and curd rice citrous fruits every day causes the development of pashanaghata sopha.

Karmavipaka of sopha is that it results due to sin of wrong deeds of previous birth. He advocates daiva vyapasraya chikitsa i.e. worshipping god, Abhisheka and dana (giving in charity) for it to overcome the disease.

He prescribes alarkadi mahalehyam, umamaheshwarasam, and kravyadi dravakam. Duration of treatment is twice a day for eight months (longer duration).

Notes:

Pashanam is a very poisonous metallic element that has three allotropic forms; arsenic and arsenic compounds are used as herbicides and insecticides and various alloys. It is administered as medicine after proper purification.

Vranasopha:

व्रणशोफेऽतिशूलं च वेदना शीतलं ज्वरः । हिध्मा हिक्का शिरोभारः शोफः सर्वांगगोचरः ॥ ३६ ॥ तंद्रा द्युन्मीलनं चापि जडत्वं श्वास उत्कटः । अनलो हृदि सन्तापो ह्यन्नद्वेषः त्वरोचकः ॥ ३७॥

ज्वरे पुराणे शुष्केडंगे सर्वांगं शिथिलं तथा । शोफोदृतिस्तदा वातः कुक्षिभारो जडत्वकम् ॥४१॥ आध्मानं चाग्निमांद्यं च निः सत्त्वं मलबद्धकं । शोषस्तंद्रा च हृत्तापः घोषः कर्णकपालके ॥४२॥ दाहो मोहः शिरो भारः स्वरो हीनो विरूपता । पूर्वपापानुसाराच्च ज्वरशोफसमुद्भवः ॥४३॥ पूजाभिषेक दानानि कृत्वाधो मास पंचकं । लक्ष्मीनारायणं लेह्यं लक्ष्मीनारायणं रजः ॥४४॥ उमामाहेश्वरं चैव मंडूरादिरसायनं । सेवयेदनुपानैश्च द्विकालं च यथोदितैः ॥४५। लेपः कौशिकतैलस्य ज्वरशोफशान्तये

Author explains that vranasopha results because of wrong deeds of previous birth.

We find mention new formulations like Varshabhu lehyam, Kausukadi rasayanam and kravyadi dravakam for the treatment of sopha.

Jwara Sopha:

The symptoms of Jwara sopha are Purana jwara,

Suskangata, Sarvanga Sithilata (looseness and weakness of the body parts), Kukshi bhara (heaviness of the abdomen), Jadatwa (stiffness), Hyumeelana (eyes are open constantly)

This clinical condition also develops because of previous birth's sin for the cause for the disease. In this treatment Lakshminarayanaras, Lakshminarayana lehyam, Lakshminarayana churnam, manduradi rasayanam are indicated. It is to be noted god lakshminarayana named after many yogas. Many a time he named names of dieties to his formulations .

It is administered 2 times a day for five months followed by lepa of kausika tailam.

Khadga ghata Sopha:

खड्गघाते ज्वरः शीतं सर्वांगं शिथिलं तथा ॥ ४६ ॥

दारुणं च तथाशूलमाध्मानं चाग्निमांद्यकम् । अन्नद्वेषो ह्याजीर्णत्वं श्वास उत्कटवेदना ॥

Jwara, sarvanga sithilatha (Lassitude), excessive swelling in the abdomen are the important features of the khadgagata sopha. This sopha also Considered as a result of sin of previous birth. Specific lehya and Rasoushadhas are mentioned namely Dhurjati Lehyam, Vaishanavirasam, gandharvarasam, mandooradi rasayanam to cure this condition. These medicines administered twice a day for eight months.

Abhishekam, puja and danam are advised. Kausika thailam recommended for external application.

Kamila Sopha:

कामिला शोफकेताप आध्मानं चग्निमांद्यकम् । लोचने पीतवर्णे च रक्तं मूत्रं
शिरोभ्रमः ॥ ५२॥ दारुणा शोफजा पीडा जडत्वं कुक्षिभारकः । वैरूप्यं शीतलं
शीतं मंदाग्निर्मलबन्धकम् ॥५३॥ शूलं सन्तापनिसृ: सत्वे चान्नद्वेषो
ह्यरोचकः । पूर्वपापानुसाराच्च कामिला शोफसम्भवः ॥५४॥
पूजाभिषेकदानानि कृत्वा द्विर्मासपंचकम् । वर्षाभूलेह्यकं चैव
वीरविक्रमसूतकम् ॥ ५५ ॥ वैष्णवी रसकं चैव क्रव्यादरसकं तथा । सेवयेत्
कामिला शोफः विनश्येन्नात्र संशयः ॥ ५६

The word Kamila is used instead of Kamala. Its characteristic symptoms include santapa (hot sensation of the body), adhmana (distention of the abdomen), pita varna netra (yellowish discoloration of the eyes), raktavarna mutra (hematuria), severe sotha (oedema), weakness, gaurava, jadatwam . The disease also results due to sin of previous birth.

Specific (anubhuta) yogas mentioned for this ailment, which include Varshabhu (punarnava) lehyam, Veeravikramarasa, Vaishnavirasa, Kravyadiras.

These formulations are used twice a day and five months is the duration.

Sarpadasta sopha:

सर्पदष्टैः क्वचित्काले गच्छत्यपि च मानवैः । तिलतैलं राजिकाश्च तिलपिष्टं
तिलानि च ॥ ५७॥ कपित्थचूतजंबीरं मत्स्यवाराहमाषकम् । भुक्तानि
चेन्मनुष्याणां दारुणं शोफ आपतेत् ॥ ५८ ॥ मंदाग्निर्मलशोषश्च
सश्वासोऽधृतिवेदने । जडत्वं सर्व संधीनां हिध्मा शीतं च शीतलम् ॥ ५९ ॥
इत्येवं लक्षणैर्युक्तः पूर्वपापानुबन्धतः । पूजाभिषेकदानानि कृत्वा
द्विर्मासपंचकम् ॥ ६० ॥ (sarpadasta sopha)

Here the author gives reason for severe swelling in snake bite that if a person consumes Tila taila (sesamum oil), rajika, tila pisti (sesamum seed), kapitha (feronia limonia), Amra (mango) Jambira (citrs lemon), matsya (fish), varaha (pig) mamsa, masa immediately after snake bite produces severe sopha (oedema). Its important symptoms include agnimandya, dryness of the stools swasayukta vedana (dyspnea associated with pain sitanubhuti (feeling cold) jadatva and sandhi sidhilata.

Due to sin of previous birth the disease gets produced. Rasoushadhas used are Varshabhulehyam, lakshmeenarayana churnam, dhurjateerasam, and vaishnavirasam. Kausika thailam to be applied twice a day for five months. Puja (prayer by worshipping god), Abhisheka, (pouring milk etc on diety) dana are to be performed.

Gandhaka Sopha:

शुद्धिशून्यं भक्षितं चेद् गंधकं शोफसम्भवः । हिध्मा हिक्का शिरोभ्रंशहुल्लसो वमनं सदा ॥ ६३ ॥ दारुणा शोफ पीडा च ग्रहणी ह्यतिसारकः । ज्वरः पिपासा द्युत्कृष्टा गले वक्त्रे च निर्द्रवः ॥६४॥ श्वासोऽधृतिश्चानलश्च करपादं च शीतलम् । प्रलापः सुप्तिशून्यत्वमनलो नेत्रयुग्मतः ।। ६५॥ सर्वांगं पीतवर्णं स्यात् पूर्वपापानुसारतः । पूजाभिषेकदानानिकृत्वा द्विश्चाष्टमासकम् ॥ ६६ ॥ धूर्जटीलेह्यकं चैव रसं मंडूरनामकम् । क्रव्यादरसकं नित्यं सेवयेद्बुद्धिमान्नरः ॥ ६७ ॥ गंधकस्य च दोषोत्थं शोफं वै दारुणं हरेत् । (gandhaka sopha)

Sotha results due to improper purification of gandhaka. We find symptoms such as karapada seetalata (Coolness in hands and feet), atisara, jwara, and yellowish discolouration of all parts of the body. It can also be said that the term probably indicates allergic swelling developed due to smelling of poisonous substances or poisonous fragrances of some of the plants. The condition may also depict drug sensitivity reaction.

This sopha is also results due to sin of previous birth. Yogas specifically mentioned to treat this condition are dhurjati lehyam, mandurarasa, kravyadi dravakam. Observing the above pattern of prescriptions it can be presumed that one lehya, churna, one rasa, and one dravaka and one thaila pattern is generally followed in the prescription.

Duration of treatment is twice a day for eight months. Puja, abhisheka and Dana are to be followed.

Kittadi kashaya:

किट्टामलकजः क्वाथः पांडुं शोफं च कामिलाम् ॥ ६८ ॥

चिंचाकिट्टकषायश्च शोफं पांडुगदं हरेत् । kashaya prepared from mandura, amalaki is to be administered for the treatment of pandu sopha and kamala.

Important rasoushadhas used in this disease are as follows:

Sophankusa rasa; Sophamudgara rasa; Sophari rasa; agnikumara ras

Above rasoushadhas mainly contain parada, gandhaka, vatsanabha, tikshna loha, tamra etc., generally administered with sitala jala or ardraka swarasa as anupana.

Vajramandura:

सूक्ष्मवज्रवल्ल्याः समांशेन चिंचायाः क्षारतोयुतं । भक्षितं चाक्षमात्रं तु
ह्यसाध्य श्वयथुं जयेत् ॥ ८८ ॥ चूर्णित मंडूरं गोमूत्रे पाचयेद्दिनम् ॥ ८७ ।

तिंत्रिण्या कणया युक्तं मंडूरं सेवयेद् भिषक् । मंडलं हरति क्षिप्रं शोफ
पांडुक्षयादिकम् ॥८९॥

In this, fine powder of mandura is boiled in gomutra for 1 day after swanga sitala this material is to be dried and administered with equal quantity of asthisrinkhala (cissus quadrangularis) cinca kshara (alkali).

Tintrini mandura: Powder of cinca and pippali with mandura bhasma is to be administered for 1 mandala. The dose is given as aksha pramana (12grams).

Notes :

Mandur Bhasma also spelled as Mandoor Bhasma comprising of calcined iron and mainly indicated for the purpose of treating and managing iron deficiency anemia.

Pathya (beneficiary diet) : Godhuma, patola, amalaki punarnava, draksha, candana etc. madhu are considered beneficial.

Apathya (Harmful diet) :

Dadhi, pungent items, sour items, vidahi (causing burning ensation in the chest) and tila are considered harmful.

The following are the rasoushdas are the new formulations by the author.

1) sophankusarasam (sheets of tamra, rasam, gandhakam)
2) Sopha mudgara rasam (rasam, gandhakam, tamrabhasma, pathya, valuka guggulu).
3) Sopharirasam (Rasam, gandhaka, tamrabhasma, tamra)
4) Rasabhupathi (rasam, gandhakam vatsanabhi, teekshnam, tamra)

Vatavyadhi:

देवानां ब्राह्मणानां वा धनापहरणात्तथा । स्वामिद्रोहाद्वातरोगी भवेदस्यापि
निष्कृतिः ॥ (कार्येति शेषः) ॥

गुरुप्रत्यर्थितां यातो वातरोगी भवेन्नरः । नाममंत्रेण कुर्वीत जपं होमं च शांतये ॥ ३ ॥

विषूचिका वांति विदाहकाश्च ज्वरोऽतितृष्णाप्यतिसारकश्च । पित्तं च मूर्छा भ्रमणं विकारो धूमाख्यवातं तु वदंति तद्ज्ञाः ॥ १०५ ।

।वदेज्ज्वरविदाहविकारकंपदेहातिदुःखगतिपीडितवांतिजुष्टम् ।शूष्कांगकं च शिरसो भ्रमणं क्षुताढ्यं निष्ठीवनं समलरोधनकुक्षिदाहम् ।। १०७ ।देहशोफो ज्वरः कार्यं कासश्च ह्यल्पभाषिता । देहस्थौल्यं च यत्रैतत् कफवातस्य लक्षणम् ॥ परस्यात्कटतायुतम् शिरः शूलं रक्तनेत्रं विधूमं वातकं विदुः ॥ १०६

जिह्वाग्र बंधनं दोषज्वरस्तृष्णापरिभ्रमः । मूकता बधिरत्वं च जिह्वांगानिललक्षणम् ॥ १०९ ॥

संतापो दृष्टिहैन्यं च शिरोभ्रमण कंपने । ज्वरश्च कंठतोदश्च स्कंधवातस्य लक्षणम् ॥ ११० ॥

दाहश्शुष्कांगशोफश्च तंद्रा निद्रामतिभ्रमः । ज्वरस्तृष्णाविकारश्च वातकंधरलक्षणम् ॥ १११ ॥

मोहोऽगघाततंद्रे च ज्वरशूलं च कंपनम् । अक्षिशूलं कर्णशूलं शिरःशूलं गुदे च रुक् ॥ ११२ ॥

कटिज्वरः पांडुश्च हिक्क च नासिका रक्तसंसुतिः ॥ ११३ ॥

देहकंडूः शिरः कंडूः कासः स्यान्मधुवातके ।

शूलं पादशूलं पादवातस्य लक्षणम् ।

ज्वरश्च वह्निमांद्यं च निद्राभंगविदाहकौ ।। ११४॥ देहावरोधनं दुःखं शिरोभंगः परिभ्रमः । अतिमूर्छातिशीतं च वस्तिवातस्य लक्षणम् ॥ ११५ ॥

क्षुतं शरीरदौर्बल्यमन्नद्वेषो विकारिता । अग्निमांद्यं ज्वरस्तृष्णा क्षुतवातस्य लक्षणम् ॥ ११६ ॥

देहः पांदुश्च शुष्कश्च निद्रानाशः शिरो व्यथा। वांतिर्हिक्का च विदेहः पांदुश्च शुष्कश्च निद्रानाशः शिरो व्यथा। वांतिर्हिक्का च विस्फोटशृंखलावातलक्षणम् ॥ १: ७॥ स्फोदेहस्य स्फटितं पुंसामंगवैकल्य पीडने। देहशोफो नेत्रशूलं स्नायुवातस्य लक्षणम्।। १११ ।। टशृंखलावातलक्षणम्॥ १: ७॥

स्खलनं वातशोफौ च करपाद विदाहकौ। स्वेदो मूर्छाभ्रमस्तृष्णा गृध्रवातस्य लक्षणम्॥ १२स्खलनं मेढ्रपायवोश्च विदाहः करपादयोः। स्वेदो मूर्छाभ्रमस्तृणा पांशुवातस्य लक्षणम्॥ १२१॥० ॥

स्खलनं मेढ्रपायवोश्च विदाहः करपादयोः। स्वेदो मूर्छाभ्रमस्तृ णा पांशुवातस्य लक्षणम्॥ १२१॥

शुक्रस्य पुंस्त्वहैन्यं च विदाहं च विकारिता। अंतर्वायुप्रकोपश्च शुक्रवातस्य लक्षणम्॥ १२अंगमर्दो ज्वरः कंपो पिपासा गुरुगात्रता। शिरस्तोदोंऽग्नि तापश्च सूतिकावातलक्षणम्॥ ४॥

Notes:

Vata is one among the three Doshas. It is a prime driving force behind all the body activities. The activities of Pitta and Kapha, dhatus (tissues) and malas (excreta) are all dependent on Vata.

Vata is a Tantra (formula), which runs the Tantra (machine) of our body. Vata also controls the mind, senses and perception. When this Vata gets disturbed it drives the body crazy. It disturbs all the events in the body and causes many sorts of damages and diseases. Vata broadly can be described as the nervous system which is the major controlling, regulatory and communicating system in the body. it is the center of all mental activity including thought, learning and memory. All these functions are done when vata is under normal conditions. The characteristics of normal vata, and the characteristics when vata vitiated i.e in aggravated state are given by acharyas like what are the causes that aggravated and also what regimen shold be adopted in treating vata dosha accordingly physicians follow to diagnose and treat.

In vaidyacintamani with reference to vata vyadhi nidana (causative factors), Samprapti (development process of disease) and other classification are similar to Madhavanidana, verses also taken from the text Madhavanidana. Apart from those mentioned in Madhavanidana author has added up many vatavyadhi, which deserve special mention.

In vata prakaranam we also get karma vipaka and and to santi mentioned just as any other disease (described earlier)

We also get exclusive pacifying measures for dhanurvata (tetanic convulsions), pakshavata and raktavata, vatarakta (gout) we also find Jyotissastra abhipraya.

Importance of Vayu: For longevity and strength vata is considered essential .It regulates the bodily functions. The entire world is regulated by vayu, when it get vitiated itproduces eighty types of diseases. It is the king and considered god itself.

Its main symptoms when deranged include contraction in body parts, stiffness, pain in the joints, rigidity at limbs, back, neck and head, insomnia, tremors, etc. The basic treatment modalities include snehana (intake of unctuous substances like oil etc. and swedana (sweating), vasti and virechana.

Causative factors (nidana) of vata roga: Excessive indulgence of excessive dry, cold food, keeping awake at nights, excessive discharge of dosas and blood from the body during sodhana kriya, long distance walk, grief, trauma to vital organs etc., causes the channels in the body to become empty which later gets filled with vitiated vata and produces different diseases afflicting one or more parts of the body.

In purva rupa (premonitory symptoms) of vataroga the symptoms of vataroga appear in mild form.

Symptoms: Contracture of the body parts, pain all over the body, breaking pain in the bones, wasting of the bodily parts. Frequent convulsion and debility are common symptoms of aggravated vata.

The following is the anatomical description of organs which fecilitates in understanding of the movement of dosa and also their original places. Firstly he describes about Kosta.

Kostha (digestive system) consists of 8 parts. Amasaya, agnyasaya, pakvasaya mutrasaya, raktasaya, hridaya, unduka, and pupphusa are considered as kostha.

Amasaya is situated in between nabhi (umbilicus) and sthana (breast). If aggravated vata if lodged in pakwasaya (between large intestine and rectum).

Likewise he gives description about symptoms sarvanga vata i.e., if aggravated vata when moves into the entirebody body causes following abnormalities. When distributed througout the body it produces tremors splitting and other types of pain etc.

If aggravated vata enters guda (rectum) causes distensionof the abdomen pain in the calves mutra sarkara (uyrinary gravel). Pain in the leg and back produced. If vata enters sensory organs it causes loss of its function. Person loses tactile sensation i.e inability to perceive hot, cold soft, and hardness of given substances .When vata vitiated it produces jrimba, alasya (laziness) pralapa (delirium) etc.If situated in skin causes dryness, cracks, loss of sensation etc. If aggravated vata locates in rakta causes increased feeling of heat, discolouration and severe pain .If located in mamsa and medas it produces feeling of heaviness of the body extreme exhaustion and pain

In medogata vata, vata causes granthi and vrana associated with manda pida (slight pain) . If located in bone aggravated vata causes pain in bones and joints. Continuous pain loss of strength. In majja gata vata it causes constant splitting pain in the body. In sukra gata vata there will be premature or delayed ejaculationof semen and also cause foetal abnormalities.

In snayu gata vata it causes convulsions and tremors

He also describes the symptoms if pitta kaphavrta prana vayu lakshana, pittakaphavrita udanavayu lakshana pitta kaphavrta samana vayu lakshana, pitta kaphavrita apanavayu (when apanavayu obstructed by pitta and kapha) lakshana, pitt akaphavrita vyana vayu lakshana separately.

Notes:

The word Avarana means obstruction to the normal gati of vata. Vata dosha is the gatyatmak dravya (moving substance) within the body. Hence its normal gati is hampered or vitiated, thus vata becomes avrutta. The course of vata gets enclosed either by the other two doshas, or any of the seven dhatus or the three malas result in Avarana. Produces symptoms depending on the site of avarana and the treatment also depicted depending on the site of avarana.

In Ayurveda eighty types vata vyadhis are described. The symptoms, which are added by the author, are given under.

Name of Vatavyadhi	Added important Symptoms by the author
Dhumavata lakshana Vidhumavata Ekangavata	Visuchi, vanti, vidaha, ratavarna netra, weakness in walking,, constipation.
Kaphavata Jihwangavata	Mukatwam (dumbness), Jihwangabandhanam (tongue drawn inside)
Skandhavata	Drustiheena
Kandharavata	Matibhrama
Padavata	He has mentioned this disorder apart from pada daha and pada harsa.
Madhuvata	Bleeding per nose and itching sensation in body and specially head.
Vastivata	Atimurcha, sirobhangha and paribhrama. Intense coolness of the body.
Kshutavata	Sneezing
Shrunkhalavata	Paleness of the body, hiccups.
Visphotavata	(Excessive Ver tigo) Ateeva sirobhrama) along with visphota
Pamsuvata	Secretions from anus and penis.
Skhalana vata	Coolness of body soon after sexual intercourse and ejaculation
Suklavata	Semen taking different route
Sootikavata	Pains in all over the body heaviness and swelling in the body.
Twagvata	Brittlessness and cracking of the body parts.
Bhogavata	Burning sensation, pain in the eyes, head

	and all over the body
Kikkisavata	Pain around the waist, head feet and nose.
Kativata	Throbbing pain around the waist anger, Prattle (Psychological symptom)
Malabaddhavata	Pain in the chest and thighs, obstruction in the passage of urine. Shivering of head.
Mootrabaddha vata	Lacking luster of the body, burning sensation while passing urine.
Urusthambha vata	Stiffness of thighs Nakha shula (pain in the nails vomiting of the blood.
Uruvata	Paleness of the body, urine will be white and frothy (symptoms do not relate to Uru)
Timira vata	Perception is lost just as the skin of elephant
Kampa vata	Shivering of hands and feet Matiksheena depressed and Dukhita mournful.
Bahu Kampa vata	Shaking of one hand, immensely mournful
Seetavata	Coolness of the body
Siravata	Pain in all over the body. Body attaining either white or yellowish discolouration of the body.
Nayanavata	Throbbing of eye balls, burning sensation of the eyes, phirangi bark powder along with rasakarpoora
Nasavata	Mahabhayam (Excess of fear) .Bleeding per nose.
Mukhavata	Dyspnoea, discharge of sputum from mouth and nose
Udaravata	Udarashula Bahukampa
Kukshivata	Nabhishula, Kukshishula Note: Udaram, kukshishula and nabhi shula accurately differentiated.
Amlavata	Aruchi, eructations, indigestion identical with the symptoms of amlapitta.

Vilomavata	Atitandra (excess of sleepiness pain in the eyes)
Dhanurvata	Body bending like bow appearing like dead body (Mrutyutulya)
Pakshaghata Vayu	Only half of the body having the pain sensation. Pain all over the body continuously through day and night. Author has described Pakshavadha vata earlier were loss of movement is the main feature, here there is loss of sensation. This might made him to describe as a separate vata disorder. It can be thought the author having profound practical knowledge, and with vast knowledge in ayurvedic classics was in a position to name new disorders along with their symptoms and has courage enough to add up to the text.
Ardhanga vata	Ardhanga bhahu Kampa (Stiffness of half of the body) Hridayagni (burning sensation of the stomach)
Parshva vata	Half of the portion of the body becomes cool, becoming unmada. Author while describing the disorders of vata roga many of psychological symptoms are also described i.e. Hasyam, unmadam etc. He made distinction between pakshavadha, pakshaghata, Ardhangavata and paksha vata.
Agnivata	The body is felt as though burnt by fire, lacking luster.
Adhyavata	Shironetra bhrama, pada shula karma shula
Sushka vata	Paleness of the body, Kampa, bhrama, tapa
Supta vata	Bhaya, chitta vikara, krodha fear disorder in thinking

Sandhivata	Feeling as if body is applied with scented ointment Angasandhishu peeda – (pain in the body and joints) Romaharsha (Horripilation)
Sadhyavata	Romaharsha, Sirashula and bhramana bhadhiryam (deafness) Ajnanam (lack of knowledge) Note: Sadhya generally indicative good prognosis of disease then naming, as sadhya to a disorder requires further study.
Sirovata	Sirovata, Horicehula, Romaharsha, daha sarvanga and netra
Swara heenavata	Swaraheena (feeble voice) Karma shula (Pain in the ear)
Rakta vata	Deha kampana, Rakta vanti, deha kanti hara Raktavanti (colloquial terminology for hematemesis).
Ksheena vata	Deha Ksheenata (depletion) Divaratrautacha Visista nidra (not getting sleep throughout day & night)
Khanjavata	Day time sleep but sleeplessness at night, Nischesta (unconsciousness)
Kalavata	Sareera Panduta, Rakta netrata, Asya Vaivarnya, Krishna Jihwha Note: colours.
Avayavangavata	Non passage (obstruction) of stools and urine sleeplessness
Sthyanavata	Mahavatam, Divaratrau shula- (colic day & night) Sadanirasanam (not having appetite at any time) Note: He has used the word mahavatam to express the intensity.

Gulbha vata	Katidesecha Tapanam (burning sensation around the waist)
Angulee vata	Burning sensation of the fingers, folding of the fingers
Januvata	Janu suskatvam
Jangha vata	Bheetam bheetam (extremely fearful) Nireekshanam (stared looking without winking)
Asthi vata	Srotretibadhiratwam (deafness in excess)
Kaka vata	Hasta pada kampa, Sirobhramanam
Bhramana vata	Bhramana, Angasopha
Pangu vata	Gatibhanga
Danda vata	Swapika udaragandhana (smells as if applied gandha over the body) stiffness of the body. Stifness of the body
Mandavata	Paleness of the body, Bhrama (giddiness)
Kosta vata	Heena vata
Gulmavata	Ajeerti (colloquial word) Bhojane Bhango (dislike for food)
Majja vata	Sarvanga shotha (swelling all over the body)
Kshata vata	Nabhi shulam (pain in the cumblicus) Kukshishulam (pain in the gesture regious)
Vasa vata	Gatra, netrasopha (swelling of the body and eyes) Nasa shulam
Anuvata	Kubjarupa (dwarfism) Gatedbhango (inability for walking)
Dadhi vata	Akshi shulam, karna shulam, Nasa shulam (pain in eyes, ears and nose)
Karina vata	Maha shulena peedanam (severe pain in the ear)

	Ahoratramcha dukham (Mourning day & night)
Badhira vata	Deafness
	srotradhwani (Tinnitus of the ear)
	Note: Both the above conditions bears slight difference
Unmada vata	Bhutavesa Vikara Krit unmata (insanity) digambara (nude)
Urdhwavata	Malabaddham (constipation)
	Annam Ksheenam (dislike for food)
Amavata	Paleness of the body and urine
	Yellowish discolouration of the eyes.
	Vomiting – warm sensation of the body.
	Note: It is strange to note that the inclusion of Amavata in vataroga. Even then above symptoms does not match with Amavata mentioned in Ayurvedic texts. @

While describing about the treatment of vata vyadhi he advocates different treatment depending on the location of vata i.e kostha, amasaya gata and pakwasayagata.

In kostha gata vata, apart from snehana and swedana kindling of digestive fire by administering dipana dravyas like citraka, yavakshara administered with takra, dadhi, manda (scum of boiled rice) . Later drinking abundant quantity of milk is advocated.

In Amasayagata vata patient should take dipana, pacana dravya before food And inducing vamana, tikshna virecana, then food prepared with mudga, puranashali dhanya (old shali rice) are advocated as pathya. .

In pakwashaya gata vata administering of agnidipaka aushadhi (digestant drugs) and also to adopt treatment procedures of udavarta (Upward or backward or reverse movement of Vata Dosha) indicated. Usually measures to overcome obstruction to the normal pathway of Vata i.e Sneha virecana, vasti sodhana followed by lavanayukta bhojana are indicated. We get extensive descriptions of vata chikitsa depending on various types of vata dusti as follows.eg, sarvanga vata cikitsa (vata vitiation in entire body), gudastita vata chikitsa (deranged vata located rectum and anal region), srotadi gata vata chikitsa (deranged vayu spread in channels) . And also we find vata treatment depending on the deranged vata symptoms like jhrimba vatachikitsa, pralapaka vatachikitsa, rasagyana vata (loss of taste), supti (Loss of sensation) vata cikitsa, dhatu gata vata chikitsa, snayu gata vata chikitsa, sandhigata Deranged vata located in joints. Vata chikitsa in pitta kaphasrita vata pitta hara treatment and incase of vatakaphsrita vata, vatakaphara treatment is advised.

Following are the formulations to rectify deranged vata:

Maharasnadi kashaya, mahabaladi kashaya, masadi kashaya, kapikachvadi kashay, rasnadi kashaya, swachanda bhairavarasa, sameerapannaga rasa, vataraksha rasa, vatari rasa sameera gajakesarirasa, mritasanjeevani rasa vatagajankusa rasa, vyadhi gajakesari rasa, surya prabha gutika, laghu vata vidhwamsini vati vatavidhwamsini rasa, rasendra chintamani, kalakanthaka rasa trugunakhya rasa, vatankusha rasa, vatamudgarasrasa, vatakesari rasa, vijaya bhairava rasa (exclusively indicated in kampavata), mukhavata chaturmmukharasa (exclusively indicated in mukhavata), kalagnirudra rasa indicated eighty vata rogas.

kalakantharasa exclusively indicated in pakshaghata. kanaka sundararasa (in supti vata), raktavatantaka rasa (for raktavata), vatavajra rasa (for khanjavata), vatanulomana rasa (for styana vata) .

Each rasoushadha is preapared targeting one specific vata disease is his speciality. The following are rasoushadhas are administered in following specific vata disease given in bracket.

Prana vallabha rasa (gulphavata), lakshmivilarasa (for jangha vata), Vijaya bhairavirasa, kalakantaka rasa (for mandavata), trivikrama rasa for gulma vata hingwadi churna, rasnadi churna, bakuchyadi churna, pathyadi guggulu sadasiti guggulu, viswadya guggulu (for vajikarana) .Among tailas ketakadi taila, sarja taila, masadi taila, maha vishagarbha taila, prasarini taila, satavari narayana taila, vishagarbha taila, vyaghri taila, mahabaladi taila, satavari taila, chandanadi taila, rasna putika tailam, bala tailam, visatinduka tailam, arkadi tailam are commonly used. Erandaputapaka, rasonapaka, kuberapaka, lasunapaka pippalyadi gutika, prabhavati gutika

Pancanana kalpa for snayu vata, bharangi nasya, kashmaryadi nasya, kumkumadi nasya, trikatukadi nasya are some of the popular formulations mentioned by the author in the treatment of vata vyadhi.

Gandamala: Author after mentioning of karmavipaka of gandamala, he mentions that because of krimi four varieties of diseases emerge from granthi. If they take origin from hridaya, it is known as hridaya gandamala. If takes origin from kantha it is known as kantha gandamala, kapola gandamala is that which takes origin from skull, if the origin is kapola it is known as kapola gandamala. Uttamnga gandamala occurs nearby head.

Notes: *Gandamala is a pathological condition, which presents as swelling in the neck (cervical lymphadenopathy). While Galaganda (goiter) is a single swelling occurring on the side of the neck, gandamala is a series of similar swellings in the neck, which looks like a garland of swellings.*

Description of gandamala in Vaidyacintamani: According to him it is equal to the size of fruits of karkandu (large type of badara) badara, amalaki, swellings will appear in kaksa, skanda, manya, gala vaksana is called gandamala. This condition develops due to vitiation of kapha and is chronic in nature and soft in consistency.

Ulcer formation, producing secretions with foul smell are the complications. Its important formulations are gandamala kashaya, kancanaradi kashaya and these formulations mainly consists of kanchanara twak and shuddha guggulu.

Gandamala kandana rasa and gandhakadi lepa, mundimula lepa, bhallatakadi lepa are mentioned for external application. Nepala patradi lepa, kanchanara guggulu (tripahala and kanchanara twak important ingredients), ajamodadi tailam, nirgundi tailam and gunjadi tailam are other important formulations for gandamala.

Disease as a cause to produce other disease:

Author mention some of the diseases are causative factors for other disease. Eg., psoriasis a skin disorder causing arthritis a joint disease. We find disease causing disease references in brichetrayee too but not in manner as mentioned in vaidyachintamani. The following are some of the examples.

Disease	**Causing the disease**
Jwara santapa	Raktapitta
Raktapitta	Jwara
Jwara and rakta pitta	Swasa
Pleecha Vriddhi	Jathara
Arsas	Udara, gulmaroga
Diwaspna	Pratisyaya
Pratisyaya	Kasa
Kasa	dhatukshaya

VISHA PRAKARANAM

The following information available on poisions in Vaidya chintamani.

Krtrima visa: The poison of different poisonous animals enter into our body system through nails, teeth and by mixing lehya, churna, then slowly that poison after fifteen days are one month produces following diseases viz: jadatha, kasa, swasa, balaksaya, rakta srava, jwara, sotha,, pitavarna of netra, and it is called kritrima visa .

To cure this condition he prescribes exclusive rasoushadha namely Bhima rudra rasa with important ingredients like swarna, suddha parada, swarnamakshika, suddha gandhaka (3parts) . Another prescription by name satyadi yoga indicated in kritrima visa. Sati, puskaramula is to be cooked with kapota pitta and administered with cold water.

Another formulation by name abhayadi ghrta with important ingredients haritaki, bhunimabha patra goghrta etc, indicated in all types of visa dosa . Another important yoga by name sarpakshi yoga indicated all types of visa dosa. In this all parts of Sarpakshi (polygonum plebium) are collected and made into coarse powder and kashaya is prepared and administered.

समूलपत्रां सर्पाक्षीं जलेन क्वथितां पिबेत् ।। ८ ।। नरमूत्रैश्च वा पिष्टां
पिबेत्सर्वगदापहम्।

Sarpakshi is to be triturated with human urine and administered in all types of visa.

Aswini kalpa is also administered for all kinds of visa. Its important ingredints are nyagrodha, haridra, kusta, griha dhuma and tanduliya mula each taken 1part.

In vaidya chintamani there is no classification of sthavara Jangama visha and also he did not follow the traditional order of the classification and also lacks other theoretic details in the book. But the chapter involves much of prescriptions to overcome the poisonous effects of the animals and substances. He also discusses an instant cure for poison of bhallataka in the form of application prepared from sirisha, meghanadham, added with navaneetam is surprising. There is mention of treatment of raby dog. Guda, tila, arka dugdha are mixed together and applied in the form of lepa. He describes single drug formulations such as apamarga roots kshara 12 grams mixing with honey used for internal administration followed by lepa over the bite area of mad dog and fox bite.

We also find formulation for an instant relief from rat bite as follows:

1) Silajitu, Talakam, kustam given mardana in nirgundirasa relieves rat bite poison .
2) Consuming cinchaphala along with gruhadhumam taken along with old ghee cures rat bite poison.
3) Taking of Sirisha, vatsanabhi given maceration of seeto daka cures rate bite poison immediately.
4) Nagaram macerated with water and administered as nasya cures it.
5) Vatsanabhi and Saindhava lavana macerated together and administered as drink.
6) Arka, dhattura mulam macerated with water and administered as drink.

Likewise we get reference for the treatment for the poison of scorpion.

Note the following simple formulation is contributed by him.

Kakajangha mula triturated in kanjika. (or) Applying the paste of Kakajangha i.e both internally and externally.

Prabhavati vati: Its important ingredients include haridra, nimba, pippali musta, vidanga, haritaki, patha etc., is tirtuarated in gomutra are prepared in to vati and administered. It is administered with different anupana in different types of visa as follows.

Above formulation used with the following anupana	Clinical Condition
Butter Milk	Snake bite
Chandana	Heavy bleeding
Kakmachiras	timira
Neelini ras	bleeding
Jaggery	vata diseases
Bhringaraja swaras	Burning sensation of the head
Cow's urine	Pleeha roga
Goats milk	Rajayakshma

Above formulation also administered in the form of lepanam, anjanam. Above formulation added with gomutra or arka and applied to relieve from scorpion bite. If prepared with kanda rasa and applied as anjana relieves from eye diseases. In the text vaidyachintamani describing about visha and prati visha it is presented in the form of stanzas. The stanzas are presented as poem written in seesa pattern of chandas. It posses peculiar rhythm. Probabaly they sung in the form of songs amidist the rural public so that they could understand simple treatments thus accrued the benefits of the medicine.

There is description of the symptoms of snake bite. We find the description of putrajeevi drug .He advocates application of the pulp of putrajeevi drug by macerating with water on the snake bitten place.

And also, author emphasizes taking of putrajeevirasa in the dose of niska every day so as to relieve from the bad effects of all poisonous serpents.

The treatment of serpent poisons are mainly comprised of either single or two drugs which are very simple and also used in the form of internal administration, anjana, lepa etc.

Drug	Clinical Condition
Pulp of putrajeevi (lepana)	All types of poision
Putra Jeevi rasa (Internal administration)	All types of poision
Musali tankan	All types of poision
Katuka and Musalee rasa	All types of poision
Langalee kanda rasa (narya)	All types of poision
Root of arka (internal administration)	All types of poision
Tankan macerated with water	All types of poision
Kashaya cow's milk added with rajani	All types of poision
Haridra either with gomutra or Human urine or purana ghrita	All types of poision
Panchanga of aswagandha macerated in goats urine (lepana)	All types of poision
Karkatamula (Lepana)	All types of poision

Among the seeds, he has given importance to Alabu beeja, karanja beeja, kusataki beeja, sireesha beeja advised to be macerated either of them in Cow's urine and also taken them along with cow's urine. Administered in all types of poison. In another formula he advise the drugs to be macerated in goats urine and also advises to take them along with goats urine. In kalakuta visa.

It is mentioned that snake bite if taken place in krittika, mula, makha, visakha, bharani, arudra nakshatra such patients will die. He gives names for serpents depending on the day of week it bites.

1) He advocates different treatments depending on the day it bites.
2) He advocates different mantras to chant depending on the day of serpent bite. Some of the examples are given below.

SNAKE BITTEN DAY	NAME PUT AS
On Sunday	Ananta
on Tuesday	Karkotaka
on Wednesday	Garkotaka
on Thursday	Padmaka
on Friday	Mahapadmaka
on saturday	----------

SUDDHIPRAKARANAM

In suddhiprakaranam we find essential information about Rasasastra. Rasashastra is a branch of Ayurveda pharmaceutics specially dealing with the minerals, metals, precious stones, certain poisonous herbs and their processing. Rasashastra the science of mercury has enriched Indian pharmacopoeia by adding innumerable herbo-mineral formularies. Number of elements and minerals has been included in the form Rasaushadhis. Rasashastra highlighted the therapeutic efficacy of these Rasaushadhi is to cure the ailments and rejuvenate the body.

In modern term, the study and practice of rasatantra is referred as rasavidya (alchemy) . Rasa ausadhis are known as metallic preparation, which includes bhasma and sindoora. Description about Metals like gold, silver, copper, lead, tin and iron, sand, lime and minerals like red arsenic, germs, salts and red chalk are given in the text vaidyacintamani.

MINERALS – The materials are very potent in eliminating diseases and also for rejuvenation purposes, mineral based products are known as Rasaushadhis. Minerals perform several vital functions, which are absolutely essential for the very existence of organism, neuro muscular stability, fluid balance and osmotic regulation. Certain minerals are integral components of biologically important compounds such as Haemoglobin. Sulphur is present in Thiamine, Biotin, Lipoic acid and co- enzyme. A several minerals participate as co-factors for enzymes in metabolism.

Calcium is the main element, which is present in bhasma of Sudhavarga dravya.

METALS –

Almost all metals are derived from ores, which means concentrations of appropriate minerals accessibly situated at or near the earth surface. The sanskrit word Loha derived from a root"Luha" meaning to pull. Thus ores, from which the metals are extracted were known as Loha.If doshas are ksheena they are boosted by samanguna, aggravated doshas are evacuated this is chikistasiddhanta. The same should be adopted with Rasaushadhis.Lohabhasma is given in Panduroga.

In vaidya cintamani text relating to rasasastra and yantras have been described into two separate chapters. Author follows the principle of Rasaratna Samuchaya with respect to suddhi of saptadhatu (swarna rajata,, pittala, naga, vanga, tiksana loha are considered as sapta dhatu) Swarna, rajata, tamra and pittala are collected and made into thin sheets and heated into red hot state then quenched in taila, takra, kanji, gomutra, kulatha kwatha simultaneously three times in each liquid.

Notes: *Suvarna (gold), rajata (silver), tamra (copper), loha (iron) are considered as sudha lohas (found in their pure form in nature) naga (lead), vanga (tin) are puti lohas Puti means putrified smell. Whatever metals emit putrified smell on heating is called puti loha alteration of colour seen in these lohas on exposure to atmposphere. Pittala (brass), kamsya (bronze) vartaloha are known as misra loha (combination of more than 2 metals are called misra loha) . Apart from nine lohas mandura/lohakitta (rusted iron) is also described.*

Suvarna Suddhi: Drugs namely valmika mrittika grhadhuma (kitchen smoke), gairika (red ochre), istika (brick powder), saindhava lavana (rock salt), jambira (citrous lemon), kanji (sour gruel) kantaka vedhi swarna patra (Thin gold sheets) triturated in jambira swarasa and kanji simultaneously then applied over kantaka vedhi swarna patra and dried, then this material is kept in earthen pot, then puta is given with 30 cow dung cakes. Like this 7 puta are repearted in unairy places. If swarna matra is more, than number of cow dung cakes to be increased. After this swarna patra is collected then swedana is done with kanji, nimbuswarasa, takra, dugdha, simultaneously five times in each liquid and then swarna should be cleaned by water.

In Vaidyachintamani while describing about Swarna bhasma, he mentions that mercury and sulphur should be taken in equal quantity and made into Kajjali (combination of mercury with sulfur in varying proportions) by giving mardana in Kanchanararasa. He also advocates that langalee, Jwalamukhee and manasila can also be used to give mardana to swarna sheets.

We also note a new concept in the process of swarna bhasma that the sheets of gold are applied with paravata or kukkuta mala and are placed on gandhaka churna in an earthen pot and again over the the swarna patra another layer of suddha gandhaka churna is poured taking gandhaka equal to the quantity and sandhi bandhana (earthen pots combined together by applying a greasy substance) is done. There after with five dung cakes kukkuta puta is given, like this nine putas are to be repeated, then in tenth puta thirty cow dungs are used there after swarnabhasma is obtained.

Notes:

For the purpose of purification and incineration, specific amount of heat is given to metals and minerals. This is quantified as Puta. In Rasashastra, Puta involves specific quantity of fuel in specific area of pit where heating process is carried out by keeping dung cakes.

The name Bhasma is generally applied to all metallic and non metallic substances that are subjected to the process of incineration and reduction into ash. Here it is applied to the scientific basis for ayurvedic therapies metals, minerals, and animal products that are, by special processes, calcinated in closed crucibles in pits with cow dung cakes (puttam) . As a result of different stages of processing techniques like shodhana (which involves roasting, with addition of herbal juices and continuous stirring) and marana which involves bhavana (wet trituration) and puta system of heating, the particle size reduces significantly, which may facilitate absorption and assimilation of the drug into the body system.

Thus formed swarnabhasma administered in different diseases with mere change of anupana. It is as follows

मत्स्यपित्तस्य योगेन स्वर्णं तत्काल दाहजित् । भृंगयोगाच्च तद्दृष्यं दुग्धयोगाद्बलप्रदम् ॥२२॥

पुनर्नवायुतं नेत्रयं घृतयोगाद्रसायनम् ।
स्मृत्यादिकृद्भचायोगात्कांतिकृत्कुंकुमेनच ॥२३। (swarna bhasma anupana)

Eg. Swarna bhasma if taken with matsyapitta (bile of fish) subdues daha (burning sensation) immediately. Along with milk reduces kshaya etc. Along with bhringaraja swarna bhasma used for the purpose of vrsya (virility). Such description is not available in any other texts of Rasa sastra

Asuddha Swarna Doṣa

बलं च वीर्यं हरते नराणां रोगव्रजान् पोषयतीह काये । असौख्यमेवं च सदैव हेमापक्वं स दोषं मरणं करोति ॥ २७॥ vrddhi, Dosa prakopa, Dukhakara, Mrtyukara Adminstration of Aśuddha swarna bhasma causes Balanaśa, Virya nasa, Roga

Description about the deleterious effects of improper purification of gold is unavailable. Author adds up some more extra points to these adverse effects such as increasing of vrana and even death.

While describing apathya he opines that Kakaradi sahita Annam, mamsa, and vyanjana are to be avoided.

Roupya (silver) :

निरीक्षयामास शिवः क्रोधेन परिपूरितः ॥ २८ ॥ ।

कस्माद्विलोचनात् । अपरस्माद्वीरभद्रो गणो वह्निरिव

बिंदुर्लोचनादपतद्भुवि । तस्माद्रजतमुत्पन्नं

ज्वलन्॥ २९ ॥ Raupyautpatti

Author explains that at the time of killing tripurasura demon, god shiva got angry, during that time tears from all the threes fell down.i.e., kamsya was originated from the tears of the first eye, god virabhadra and pramada gana originated from tears of second eye, suddha rajata produced from the tears of third eye. Kritrima rajata produced by the combination of vanga and parada. Rajata is of 3 types sahaja, kritrima and khanija. Kritrima variety of rajata placed under the footwear of god rama. Khanija rajata originated and produced in himchal Pradesh.

In other books like rasarnava it is classified as sahaja, vanga vedhaja and khanija.

Roupya sodhana is done by immersing heated plates in agastya swarasa 3 times or karkotakai kanda swarasa for 7 times or drakshakwatha or cincadrava simultaneously. This is to separate nagadhatu from rajata. Likewise marana of roupya also been mentioned. Rajata bhasma is considered as best medicine to cross the roga samudra, it is mainly indicated vataja, pittaja, kaphaja vyadhi and also pliha and yakrit rogas.

The following are some of the simple formulations of Rajata bhasma administered in many diseases by changing anupana as follows.

Notes : *Anupana is that material which is consumed along with food or medicine. It can increase the palatability of the food or medicine, can improve the digestion and absorption and also act as a vehicle, which carries the drug to their target site.*

Rajata Bhasma added with sarkara to relieve daha (burning sensation).

Rajata bhasma added with Triphala churna to cure vataja and pittaja vyadhi.

Administered with trisugandha for the treatment of prameha (urinary tract diseases including diabetes).

He too has given the deleterious effects of rajata if not purified properly.

Tamra: We find the following contributions made by him with respect to tamra. They are as follows:

Origin: Author's mythological view differs with other ayurvedic texts and according to him it is due to surya tejas falling on the earth.

The eight dosas of tamra mentioned in Vaidyachintamani almost identical with Ayurveda prakasa and Rasarathansamucchaya. Author'another contribution is indicating an universal formula ie.immersing tamra in amla dravyas to purify it . Tamra which is asuddha causes complications like vannti, bhranti, klama, santapa, sula, kandu, virecana, viryanasa. To counteract these each one of the dosha tamra is subjected to suddhi separately mentioned as follows.

Eg. Vomiting one of the eight dosas gets averted by purifying it with butter, milk, oil, cow wine. Purifying tamra with vajee dugdham and godugdham prevents Glani. Likewise he has explained shuddhi for each of the eight dosas. When proper sodhana is done it becomes non toxic and becomes like nectar.

Author did not mention synonyms of tamra. The following is the general procedure of sodhana. Copper rods are made into thin sheets of copper and heated repeatedly then quenched in taila, takra gomutra in order to reduce vanti dosa .thereafter with kanji, kulkutha kashaya to reduce bhranti dosa. Later with kshira and godugha to reduce klama dosa to reduce santapa dosha sodhana done with cinaca rasa and nimbu rasa, sodhana is done with kumara swarasa dugdha, goghrta in order to reduce kandu dosha. In suranakanda rasa and in mastu sodhana reduces virecana dosha. Afterwards sodhana done with madhu, draksha rasa in order to reduce viryanasa. Hence nepala tamra heated redhot after applying them with kshira and arka kshira pancalavana quenched in the above said liquids the process is to be repeated for seven times in above mentioned each liquid. Preparation of tamra bhasma mentioned as per bhasma procedure by subjecting them to puta. It is administered in the dose of one gunja pramana. Useful in kusta, pliha, kapharoga and gulma.

Vanga (Tin) : It is of 2 types

Author gives ranga and Trapu as synonyms of vanga. It is of 2 types khanija vanga. And misraka vanga. Khanija is considered best. Misraka is not recommended for use.

Khuraka vanga is to be melted with nirgundi swarasa and haridra churna, this process has to be repeated for three times in order to get suddha vannga. Melted vanga should be poured in each of the following liquids such as mutravarga dravya, amlavarga, ksharodaka, and vajra arka kshira. This process has to be done seven times in each liquid separately.

We get jarana and marana methods of vanga described briefly. Vanga bhasma used in the treatment of kasa, swasa, abdominall lump chest wounds and prameha (polyuria) .

The following are some of the examples

Various Anupānas of Vanga bhasma in different disease conditions

कपूरेण समायुक्तं मुख दुर्गंधनाशकम् ॥ ९४ ।जातीफलैः पुष्टिकरं वंगभस्म सदा नृणाम् । तुलसीपत्रसंयुक्त प्रमेहं नाशयेद्ध्रुवम् ॥ ९५

Vangabhasma added with karpoora relieve asya durgandha, added with jatiphala churna it is nourishing, if added with tulasi churna cures meha (urinary diseases) and adding it with haridra churna reduces Raktapitta.

Vanga bhasma along with lavanga and lepana removes impotency. Vangabhasma aso been administered with Vijaya swarasa (bhang) to get the action of virya sthambhaka. It is administered with navaneeta and dugdha as anupana. Likewise we find innumerable indications given with change of anupana.

It adverse effects i.e when it is not properly purified causes kusta (skin diseases including leprosy), prameha, vatarakta (gout) and also weakness.

Naga (lead) : Naga is of 2 varieties kumara and samala. Kumara is best and suitable for bhasma. Naga is originated from the semen of vasuki (the kingof snake, which he has discharge seeing nagakanya) . While making shuddhi of naga he specially mention about Handika yantra (the mouth of one earthen pot covered with strong lid with central hole) . Before pouring melted naga the earthen pot filled with arkadugha. This process has to be repeated for 3 times.

We also find mention of the preparation of naga sindhura adding naga with rasaka churna. It is mentioned that nagabhasma provides strength equal to 100 elephants.

. In the preparation of bhasma we find lmited ingredients, manishila is used, and mostly done with the juice of betel leaf for mardana. He advocates atarushaka kasta or lohadanda for stirring. We also see the mention of aswattha and chincha in the process of bhasma 32 or 60 putas are given to make bhasma.

Loha (iron) : Author mentioning origin of lauha states that in ancient days devatas killed romila daitya during that period different types lohas produced from his body.

मुंडाच्छताधिकं तीक्ष्णं तीक्ष्णात्कांतं शताधिकम् । तसमान्मुंडं परित्यज्य तीक्ष्णं वा कान्तमुत्तमम् ॥ १

3 varieties are mentioned. They are, kanta lauha, tikshna lauha and mundalauha. Kantalauha is considered best and is 100 times powerful than the other lauha. Sodhana recommended for lauha otherwise impure lauha causes visa dosa, klama, vamana and virya dosha contrary to seven doshas mentioned in other texts (Ayurveda Prakasa) . Author mentions different type of suddhi. i.e. he advocates to apply the blood of rabbit to the foils of loha and heated then immersed in Triphala Kashaya for three times. The bark powder of chincha macerated with arka ksheera and this is applied on the foils of loha, later immersed in Triphala Kashaya after heating them for sodhana purpose.

We do not find the description of Trividha pakas of loha i.e bhanupaka, sthalipaka and putapaka in Vaidyacintamani. Author recommends Kanyarasa (kalabanda) in the process of making lohabhasma. He advocates lohabhasma in combination with rasa to treat diseases effectively. Author omits much of the information about loha but mentions routinely used procedures which have practical relevance. We find loha bhasma added in several yogas, and such references available throught the book vaidya chintamani. We find mention of amriteekarana of lauha bhasma .Lauha bhasma is added with double the quantity of triphala kashaya and triturated well, and thereafter heated over madhyamapaka. This is known as amriteekarana of lauha. This is considered efficacious to cure all diseases. It is rejuvanative, and particularly useful in improving the the blood quality. It is balya, vrsya, sukhakaraka rasayana, kantidayaka, and rupasampadakara.

Kanta bhasma: Author mentions that if taila bindu is put in container made up of kanta lauha and filled with water, the taila buindu will not spread. If hingu is put in that acontainer it destroys the smell of hingu. Neutralizes the bitterness of nimbapatra kalka (paste). Canaka which was kept in water for sometime and kept in the container of kantalauha their external layer gets burnt. For this sodhana and marana also been mentioned. He advocates pashana bhedha swaras and palasa twak separately for this purpose. Later chakrikas prepared and gajaputas are given.Like this three gajaputas are repeated in order to obtain bhasma.

Kanta sindhura: Munda Loha (Cast Iron), Teekshna Loha (Iron Turnings), and Kaanta Loha (Magnetic ore of Iron) are the three main forms of Loha. Kaanta Loha is the best therapeutically, Teekshna Loha is better, and Munda Loha is less beneficial.

Author mentioning the preparation of kanta sindhuram mentions that 1 part of sodhita kanta lauha is to be mixed with half part of the sodhita hingula and collected into khalva yantra and then triturated with kapikacchu mula swarasa for three days. Then this material collected into vajramusa (which is prepared from the red soil) and sandhi bandhana is to be done and dried. Thereafter three gajaputas are to be repeated to obtain kanta lauha sindhura with arunodaya Varna.

Kanta dhrti:

Bones of following animals such as jackal, sheep, tortoise etc., are powdered mixed with suddha silajitu, further rmixed with kanta lauha churna and heated in iron container by adding the curna of above contentes little by ittle with continuous stirring. Kantalauha becomes liquid form similar to parada. It is indicated in the form kanta lauha bhasma in combination with abhraka bhasma and is mainly indicated in malnourishment and deficiency of blood disorders. This kantabhra sindhura mentioned by God shiva to Goddess Parvati.

The following are different types of anupana using lauha bhasma.

Loha Bhasma administered with change of anupana in different diseases as follows

Lohabhasma along with ghee given in Shula; with pippalee churnam and honey in Purana jwara; added with Trikatu churnam and honey in Swasa; lohabhasma added with Nirgundee rasa administered in aseeti vataroga. Lohabhasma added with Triphala kashaya and administered in Prameha; added with Silajitu churna and administered in Mutrakrichra (difficulty in urination);

Lohabhasma added with Triphala churna and honey and administered in all diseases.

Apthya during loha bhasma administration are kushmanda, tila taila, masa, karavellaka, tikshna dravya and amla padartha.

To understand that lohabhasma prepared to the standards, the following test is performed.

Lohabhasma pariksha: Lauha bhasma mixed with madhu and ghrta and kept in silver container and heated, ones it becomes self cooled Rajata samputa (silver container) is weighed. If it becomes reduced in weight it indicates lauha bhasma not prepared properly. This lauha bhasma again processed with marana (Marana (Incineration) is an essential step to be performed on substances) procedure

Author mentions that kantabhasma possess all the properties similar to Rajata bhasma. Hence it can be replaced with rajata if kanta bhasma is not available. It appears that he has taken some of the verses from Ayurveda Prakasa and deleted much of the portion of the text and contributed by adding of his own. (Ayurveda Prakasha is one of the important ancient texts on ancient Indian Alchemy).

We find the description about tikshna loha dravana .In this devadali bhama is applied in human urine and filtered, this process is repeated for 21 times, with this obtained kshara, tikshna lauha is heated to form tikshna drava. While doing this kshara has to be added little by little (druti). Likewise gandhaka and lauha druti also is prepared.

If lauha is heated in fire it releases its impurities known as lauha kitta. Lauha kitta, which is 100 years old, considered as uttama and which is below 60 years considered as visa (poisonous).

Author also gives a detailed note on Mandura bhasma. Mentioning preparation of mandura bhasma says that Lauha kitta (sludge iron) heated with high temperature and dipped suddenly in cows urine, same process is repeated for seven times. Then sodhita mandura is produced. This is made into powder and added with 2 times of triphala kashaya and boiled till the material gets concentrated form then this material again roasted and again made into powder form, this is called mandura bhasma. It is very useful in the diseases anaemia and jaundice.

Kantalauha bhasma is nourishing and is considered 10000 times efficacious than other lauha. In non-availability of swarna or rajata kanhta lauha bhasma can be administered.

Kamsya (bronze-bell metal) : we find the description of Kamsya in Vaidya chintamani. Kamsya (bronze) is an alloy made primarly of copper and tin. Kamsya triturated with cinca patra (tamarindus indica) rasa or kulatha (vigna unquiculata) kwatha for three times to produce suddha kamsya. We get descriptions about kamsya bhasma and kamsya sindhura (added with parada and gandhaka) . Kamsya bhasma considered improving longevity and nourishing when its bhasma administered in pure form. In vaidya chintamani we find the description of pittala (alloy made of copper and zinc) . Its sodhana is also similar to kamsya.

Parada (Mercury) : Mythological origin of parada is different in vaidya chintamani when compared to rasaratna samuchaya. It is said that Lord Siva wants to give birth to Kartikeya.

स्कंदात्तारकहिंसार्थं कैलासे पार्थितः सुरैः । करुणात्मा महादेवः पार्वतीवल्लभशिवः रतौ शंभौः च्युतं रेतो गृहीतं वह्निना मुखे । क्षिप्तं तेन चतुर्दिक्षु क्षमायां तत्पृथक्-पृथक् ॥

On the plea of Devata, Mahadeva and goddess Parvati have started sexual copulation to produce skanda for the purpose of killing demon tarakasura. But due to its interruption, the ejaculated semen hurled upon the agni, but agni could not bear hence threw it in four directions. Parada which is fallen in pascima disa remained with potency and became useful for all the purposes.

We find a reference stating how parada is obtained. The girl who bathed after menarche (1st menstrual period) after getting on the horse should proceed to see the hollow pit consisting of parada. Then parada gets attracted and will rise to the surface and thus becomes available. It is mentioned that one will accrue punya (virtue) equal to that doing 100 aswamedha yoga, kotigodana (donating one crore cows) sahasra swarna dana by the vision of it. We find the mention of rasanama are almost identical with other rasa texts.

ब्रह्मज्ञानेन संयुक्तो यः पापी रसनिंदकः । । १२५ ॥ स याति नरके घोरे जन्मकोटि शतैरपि । आलापं गात्र संस्पर्शं यः कुर्याद्रसनिंदकैः ॥ २२६ ॥
याति जन्म सहस्रणि स भवेदुः खपीडितः ।

Adverse effects of Parada Ninda Even though the person is considered as Bhramhajnani (Most knowledgeble person), if he criticizes Parada, then he gets into Naraka and retains there till Satakotijanma. The people who joins with the Parada nindaka (Person who criticizes the Parada) and touches him, then that person also suffer with Dukha upto Saharsra janma.

Eight types of Parada Dosa:

उड्डीनं चापि कौटिल्यमनवर्तं च संकरम् ॥ २२७ ॥

षण्डत्वं पङ्गुकारित्वं समलत्व गुरुत्वकम् सविषत्वं च सूतस्य चाष्टदोषाः प्रकीर्तिताः ॥ २२८॥

Rasa (Pārada) contains eight types of Dosa viz : 1. Uddina dosa, 2. Kautilya dosa, Anavarta dosa, 4. Sankhara dosa, 5.

Sandatva dosa, 6. Pangu dosa, 7. Maladosa bescause of its heavy nature, 8. Visatva dosa.

It is mentioned that dosha (blemish) resulted due to blaming of parada are given. We find the mention of rasadoshastakam, which is not similar to that, mentioned in other rasasastra texts. They are uddinam, Kautilya, anavarta, sankara, sandatwa, pangu, maladosa, because of its heavy nature and savishatvam. Parada with these doshas are not to be administered else it produces diseases.

On the basis of colour it is of 4 types. Sweta parada (bramhana), Raktavarna (Kshatriya), pitavarna (vaisya), krsna varna (sudra).

He also describes Rasa mahatmya saying that Dhatu gata dosha get destroyed by sodhita parada. Parada contains thirteen varieties of dosha. Parada is so pious that brahma hatya papa, gohatya papa gets removed by mere parada darshana and parada sparsha respectively.

Rasalinga is considered one crore times better than banalinga. Adverse affects due to parada ninda are mentioned. Person who criticizes gets into naraka (hell) and retains there till satakotijanma (hundread rebirths) and even the other person who touches suffers dukha upto sahasra janma. Different diseases caused by taking asuddha parada are mentioned. It is amazing to note that he specifies what disease will emerge from which kind of dosha. Eg, uddina dosa causes shula (pain), anavarta dosha causes Bhrama, kautilya dosha causes kapala roga etc. He also mentions sapta kanchuka dosha. They are naga, vanga, mala, agni, visa, giri, capala. Administration of parada with these dosha causes diseases. i.e naga dosha causes gandamala (cervical lymphadenitis), vanga dosha causes kustha, mala dosha effects the knowledge of memory, visa dosha causes death, agnidosha causes daha and moha, giridosha causes jadya, capala dosha causes virya dosha . Hence before administration purification is mandatory.

Procedures to remove astadasa parada:

अथातः स्संप्रवक्ष्यामि दोषाष्टकनिवारणम् ॥ २४४

इष्टका रजनी चूर्णैः षोडशांशै रसस्य च । मर्दयेत्तप्तखल्वे तज्जंबीरोत्यैर्द्वैवैर्दिनम्
॥ २४५॥

कांजिके क्षालयेत्सूतं नागदोषं विमुंचति । विशालां कोलचूर्णेण वंगदोषो विनश्यति ॥ २४६॥

राजवृक्षे मलं हंति चित्रको वह्निदूषणम् । चांचल्य कृष्णधत्तूरस्त्रिफला विषनाशनम् ॥ २४७॥

कटुत्रयं गिरिं हन्तिह्यसह्याग्निंत्रिकंटकः ।

For doing samskara the quantity of parada either should be 100 pala or 50 pala or 25 pala or 12 pala or 5 pala or 1 pala. Before doing samskara one should chant rasa samskara mantra known as aghoramantra.

अघोर इति मन्त्रेण रससंस्कर पूजनम्

अमन्त्रितपदार्थानां तेजो निघ्नंन्ति भैरवाः

To over come the disorder of the rasadoshas he advocates several formulations suited for each dosha.

Notes:

Samskara, a special type of processing of mercury, apart from alleviating the blemishes, gives strength and luster to mercury.

Taptakhalwam means, Khalwa prepared either by iron or stone, and it is to be put over the pit with fire underneath produced by hard excrement of goat etc.

Astadasa Samskaras of parada:

The rasa Asstadasa samskaras are swedana, mardana, murchana, uttapana, adahpatana, tiryakpatina, urdhwapatana, bodhana, sniyamana, dipana, anuvasana, marana, jarana, sarana, pratisarana, kramana, vedhanam and sarira yoga. By tha above procedure dosa get removed thus causes purification and potentiation.

Purified parada is administered in innumerabe diseases with mere change of adding churna.

The following are some of the examples.

Eg: 1) Parada bhasma added with pippali, maricham, sonthi churnam, taken along with honey relieves kasa, swasa.

2) Parada bhasma added with haridra, sarkara relieves from rakta vikara.

3. Parada bhasma if taken along with betel leaves one can avert constipation. He was of the view that parada bhasma taken along with pippali and guduchi during night relieves one from constipation.

We find description about extracting parada from Hingula (cinnabar).

Rasa sindhura: kajjali is prepared from parada and gandhaka and fine powder of the rest of the drugs are added and mixed together then, this material is filled in glass bottle, thereafter it is placed in valuka yantra and heated with controlled temperature for 3 days continuoiusly, then aruna varna rasa sindhura is prepared.

भागो रसस्य त्रय एक भागाः गंधस्य माषः पवनाशनस्य- सम्मर्द्य गाढं सकलं सुभांडे तां कज्जलीं काचघटी निदध्यात् । (triguna gandhaka sindhura)

We also find preparation of dwiguna (adding 2 parts of gandhaka), triguna gandhaka sindhura (adding 3 parts of gandhaka) so as to potentiate gandhaka so as to make suitable to be administered in puyameha etc., diseases

Notes: *Kajjali is used as a base for Ayurvedic herbomineral medicines. It is a combination of mercury with sulfur in varying proportions. The ratio of sulfur (S) added to mercury (Hg) directly relates to the therapeutic efficacy of the compound.*

Time schedule: It is interesting note that parada bhasma should be consumed during early morning. After 2prahara (6hours) of parada bhasma sevana, pathya bhojana is to be taken and after 3 prahara (9hours) bhojana should not be taken. Food should not be taken middle of the day.

नोल्लंघयेत्रियामं तु मध्याह्ने नैव भोजयेत् ॥ ३४७ ॥ तांबूलांतर्गते सूते विड्बंधो नैव जायते । स कंणामृतया भुक्तो मलबंधं हरेन्निशि ॥ ३४८ ॥

If parada bhsma is administered with tambula patra swarasa it will not cause constipation, but administering with pippali and guduci will cure constipation. It is stressed that during the administration of parada bhasma dravya which ksara tiksna amla should be avoided, otherwise it leads to rasajirna and causes complications like shula, daha impaired intelligence etc.

Rasakarpoora:

Rasabhasma is considered as one of the rasabheda and it is called as rasakarpoora. (Rasakarpura, the mercurial preparation is chemically found chloride salt of mercury associate with trace elements). Rasakarpoora is considered amrita (nectar) cure eighty varieties of vata roga (neurological diseases), eighteen varities of kustha (skin diseases) twenty varities of prameha (ipolyuria including diabetes), bhagandhara (fistula in ano), udara (abdominal disorders etc.), and visa vhikara (disorders due to poison).

Rasakarpura is administered in the dose of gunja 125 mg with purana guda as anupana. During its administration milk, boiled rice, Tambula (piper betle) are pathya.

We find some formulations like Karpasa dala niryasa, tanduleeya rasa along with loha churna, jeeraka etc., to act like an antedote. In this section we also find lepa (application) to mitigate rasa tapa (hot flushing experience). The drugs in the formulation include dhatri, kumara, kushmanda, bhringaraja kakamachi etc.

He gives the following another formula to mitigate rasatapa. The juice of Jambu twak, triphala, bimba kumara are mixed together and taken relieve rasa tapa. It appears that the book Vaidyachintamani is the compendium of practical experiences of the author obtained while treating these diseases. We find vadya chintamani comprising of all the time tested, remedies (anubhuta chikitsa) particularly his expertise in preparation and administering of rasoushadhas in number of diseases with mere change of anupana is laudable.

During parada sevana, old rice, cows milk, ghee, cows curd, tanduliyaka are considered as pathya. Kushmanda (benincasa hispida), vartaka (brinjal) karavellaka (bitter guard), canaka (Bengal grama), kulutha ((vigna unquiculata) anupa jantu mamsa (meat of acquatic animals, alcohol etc) are considered apathya.

Gandhaka: According to mythological story, in sweta dwipa situated in ksira sagara (milk ocean) when goddess Parvati playing with her friends she had menstrual discharge. Her cloths attached with good odour has been cleaned by her friends. This rajassu (menstrual discharge) converted to gandhaka. Bali king of demons who consumed gandhaka to gain strength during samudra mathana. Because of the heat produced from the mouth of vasuki snake, the gandhaka melted and released from the body of the Bali spread all over the earth. Since then gandhaka is available on earth.

Gandhaka which s having colour and shiness similar to kapikacchu and navanita and should be mrdu, kathina, snigdha properties is best in quality.

In vaidyachintamani a different type of sodhana mentioned for Gandhaka. He mentions that milk is filled in container and mouth of this container is tied with cloth, over the cloth asuddha gandhaka is kept and over that coth and gandhaka another container is placed, sandhi bandhana is done, then kurma puta is given. Thereafter sodhita gandhaka, which is collected in the milk, is to be used as sudha gandhaka. In another procedure instead of milk kanji is used to purify sodhana. In an iron container equal quantity of ghrta and gandhaka is added and melted. Then melted gandhaka poured in by filtering cloth in another container which is already filled with milk and gandhaka. This is to be collected from milk after swanga sitala, gandhaka is cleaned with cloth and dried in sunlight.Like this same process is repeated by changing the milk every time then it is allowed for internal administration.

Remedy for complications of gandhaka: If allegic symptoms manifested through its use then it should be discontinued and the patient may be given sufficient milk mixed with ghee .It is mainly used to treat skin diseases. Gandhaka is administered in many diseases with mere change of anupana.

One sana of suddha gandhaka is mixed with triphala ghrta, bhringaraja swarasa, madhu is to be administered to improve the eye sight and also cures eye diseases and beneficial in increasing the life span. One niska of (4grams) of suddha gandhaka is given with milk for 1 month to increase saurya (valour), and virya (sperm) .

Gandhaka druti: 1 part of suddha gandhaka is to be triturated with 1/16 th part of trikatu churna and spread over on a cloth, there after varti is prepared.This varti together with thread and immersed in tila taila for 1 yama .There after varti is taken out and when varti is burned out oil is dropped and collected to other glass container.Three bindu are placed in bettle leaf and administered in parada rasa dosa. With this, the body becomes laghu. It is administered in disease like pandu, swasa etc.

ABHRAKA (biotite mica)

Origin:

पुरा वधाय वृत्रस्य वज्रिणा वज्रमुद्धृतम् ॥४०३॥

विस्फुलिंगास्ततस्तस्य गगने परिसर्पिताः । ते निपेतुर्घनध्वानाः शिखरेषु महीभृताम् ॥४०४॥

तेभ्य एव समुत्पन्नं तत्तगिरिषु चाभ्रकम् । तद्भ्रवव्रतातत्त्वमभ्रमभ्ररवोद्भवात् ॥ ४०५ ॥

गगनात्पतितं यस्मादग्गनं च ततो मतम् ।

Author explains a different mythological story; it says that, Indra in order to kill vrittasura threw his Vajrayaudha. Thus generated flash lights because of Vajrayudha fell on mountain revolving themselves with a bee like sound. Abhraka thus generated is made available in the mountains. He mentions gaganam as its synonym since it is fallen from the sky.

Notes: *Abhraka is trasluscent and lustrous mineral, easily split into thin layers Abhraka is produced in under ground with the combination of water content in 4 to 6%.*

We get typical classification of abhraka in the book Vaidyacintamani such as brahmana, kshatriya, vaisya, and sudra. Swetabhraka useful in rajata kriya, raktabhraka useful in rasayana, pitabhraka useful in suvarna kriya, krishnabhraka is useful for the purpose of roga nasaka. Hene krishnabhraka is considered as best variety for the purpose of treating different diseases.

Abhraka pariksha: Abhraka is of 4 varieties. Pinaka, naga, Manduka (dardura) and Vajra. He mentions that Pinakabhraka when heated its layers are separated. Its administration causes Skin diseases. Dardura variety of abhraka when heated breaks into pieces and jumps like a frog and this causes constipation and ultimately leads to death. Nagabhraka when heated produces hissing sound like snake and it causes bhagandhara. Vajrabhraka when heated remains unchanged hence useful to prepare abhraka bhasma considered useful in all diseases and also reduces the incidence of death.

Abhraka sodhana is done in palika yantra and kept in kosthi and heated up to it become red hot state. This abhraka is quenched in godugdha, triphala, kanji, gomutra etc 7times in each liquid, there after rubbed with hands then abhraka is taken out and washed.

Notes:

Palika yantra A round iron container with long vertical handle bend at the end is called palika yantra used for taking out oil, jarana of gandhaka etc.

Dhanyabhraka vidhi: Author mentions different kind of dhanyabhra vidhi. Sodhita abhraka mixed with $1/4^{th}$ quantity of sali dhanya and contents are made into pottali, then immersed in water and kept in for 3 days, there after pottali is rubbed. With hands and microparticles of abhraka comes out from the pottali, then the abhraka particles are collected in the earthen pot. This abhraka particles after filtering water used as dhanyabhraka.

Abhraka sindhura (bhasma) : Trituration of in liquids like bhringaraja, guduchi, tulasi, madanaphala etc then chakrika are prepared and and gajaputa is given. (With each bhavana separate gajaputa is to be given) .Thereafter abhraka sindhura or abhraka bhasma is prepared. It cures all diseses.

We find description of three methods of preparations of satapula abhraka bhasma. In this mardana of dhanyabhra for one day in each liuid like punarnavaswarasa meghanada swarasa etc is to be done and chakrika (pellets) are prepared and dried later gajaputa is to be given. There after mardana again to be done with liquids cinca swarasa, musta swarasa and thereafter chakrika are to be prepared and dried and 3 gajaputas are given. Then again mardana is to be done in kasa marda patra swarasa and five gajaputas are given. Therafter mardana is again is to be done with gomutra then chandrika are to be done and dried and five gajaputas are given. Therafter again mardana is to be done with triphala kasaya, then pellets are prepared later five gajaputas are to be given. Again mardana is to be done with nyagrodha kasaya and ten gajaputasa are to be given. Again mardana is to be done with nimbu swarasa and chakrikas are prepared given 6 gajaputa again mardana is to be done with cow milk and 3 gajaputas are to be given. Then abhraka is to be collected and again mardana is to be done and chakrika are to be prepared. Then earthen pot is to be taken and filled with arka patra then chakrika are placed and again covered woth arka patra therafter the mouth is to be joined with the mouth of another pot and joint sealed (sandhibandhana) with mud and cloth then gajaputa is to be given by the same method total 100 gajaputa are to be repeated in order to obtain red colour bhasma similar to the colour of ruby. This abhraka bhasma will be niscandrika yukta (lusterlessness) and appears like sindhura. This sataputa abhraka bhasma can be used in the preparation of all yoga. Likewise we get reference of sataputa abhraka bhasma second and third method also the number of gajaputas in second method is 35 gajaputas, followed by 25 gajaputas, followed by 25 gajaputas later 25 gajaputas are given. Later mardana is done with cow'milk and 3gajaputas are given to obtain red colour bhasma. It will be niscandrka (lusterless) and appears like sindhura. Third method also mentioned for sataputa abhraka bhasma .

त्रिफलायाः कषायस्य पलान्यादाय षोडश । गोघृतस्य पलान्यष्टौ मृताभ्रस्य पलान् दश ||४३६|| मेलयित्वा लोहपात्रे च पाचयेन्मृदुवह्निना । तदेवं जीर्णमादाय सर्वरोगेषु योजयेत् ||४३७||

There is description of abhraka amritikarana. In this 16 pala triphalakshaya, eight pala of goghrta, 10 pala abhraka bhasma are to be taken in an iron container and heated till liquid content get evaporated .This process is known as abhraka amritikarana and it is useful in all disease conditions.It is provides strength and nourishment to the body and considered to improve longevity.

While describing about abhraka marana we come across the mention number of drugs, in whose kashayas Abhraka is incinerated. It includes even vijayadrava, Vidarikanda, Kushmanda, Bhallatakarasa and draksharasa etc. Incineration with many number of kashayas for marana are not mentioned any other texts. It is as follows.

Abhraka bhasma added with Madhu and pippalee to cure 20 varieties of prameha .Abhraka bhasma added with Swarnam to cure Kshaya.Abhraka bhasma added with Roupya, hema, abhrakam lavanga, madhu to cure dhatu Vriddhi .

Abhraka bhasma added with Godugdham, sarkara to cure Pittarogam and Valeepalita. And also, Abhraka bhasma added with Vyosham along with ghrita to cure Khaya, pandu, grahani, kustu, swasa and Prameha

Dose – Vallapramana (1 valla is equal 2 masha i.e 500mg) .

He also emphasizes there is no such drug other than abhraka bhasma which can destroy Jara (old age) and mrityu (death) . Much of the information realting to abhraka is missing in his book, but we find gyst of information about rasasastra which has practical relevance is incorporated. The following items like kshara, amla, dwidala dhanya, karkati, karavellaka vrintaka, karira tilataila are prohibited during administration of abhraka bhasma.

Haratala (orpiment) :

संध्यायांनरसिंहेन हिरण्यकशिपुर्हतः । । ४५३ । ।
तच्छविसमो भूतालस्तत्कक्षालेखनाश्रितः ।

Mentioning origin of Haratala states that Hiranya kashyapa was killed in the evening time by god Narasimha during that time Haratala is produced from the body and haratala possessing similar shininess as that of hiranya kashipa body.

Among 2 varieties (Patra haratala and pinda haratala) Patra haratala considered best. Haratal is to be done sodhana to reduce adverse reactions. Its sodhana is done by keeping haratala in dola yantra for 1 yama and also swedana is done with kanji, kushmanda swarasa, and godugdha 3 days each and lastly vata ksira swedana is done for 3 days to obtain suddha haratala. To prepare bhasma suddha haratala is triturated in punarnava swarasa for 1 day .later pellets are prepared and dried. Punarnava kshara is to be placed in an earthen pot and over the kshara Haratala chakrika is kept in and covered with an earthen pot and sandhibandhana is done, then this sarava smputa is to be heated gradually and continuously for 5 days to prepare haratala bhasma. It is administered in the dose of ratti with suitable anupana. If haratal bhasma poured over the fire, there should be no smoke, a characteristic of suddha bhasma. If smoke obtained then it is considered that the bhasma is not prepared properly. It is generally administered in the dose of ½ gunja with 6 valla of khandasarkara. The following like lavana, amla dravya, katurasa dravya, usna guna dravya, atapa sevana are to be restricted.

Anjana: Anjana is said to be compound of antimony. Author puts forward a totally different classification of anjana i.e. 2 varieties, namely vamanjana and kapotanjana instead of 5 varieties found in rasatantra texts. But the description of srotonjanam and neelanjanam is available. We do not get reference of rasanjan and pushpanjana. In Caraka and susruta samhitas diferent anjanas have been referred to and used as medicine both internally and externally. For the purpose of sodhana srotanjana, sauviranjana should be cooked in triphala kashaya and Bhringa raja swarasa. For sodhana of Nilanjana etc., Nilanjana are to be made into powder form and triturated with jambira swarasa and one day dried in sun light. The nilanjana is used for all purposes.

Kaseesa (green vitriol) : Author classifies kaseesa into 2 types i.e Valuka kaseesa and pushpa kaseesa as mentioned by rasaratnakara. He considers valu kaseesa is best and did not describe about pushpa kareesa. Synonyms of kaseesa are dhatu Kaseesam, pansu Kaseesam, kesaram, Anyam, malyarasa, puspa kasisa, and netrabhusana.

Sodhana: He follows Ayurveda prakasakara and rasatarangini method i.e. by using Bringa raja swarasa (eclipta alba) as swedana dravya to get it purified.

Kaseesa guna: It appears that the verse taken from Rasaratna Samucchaya but he deletes 1st stanza, which describes about valukaseesa, but describes about puspa kaseesa. It is mostly used in switra (lucoderma), vrana (ulcer) and vata vyadhi (neurological diseass).

kasisa Bhasma: We find different mode of bhasma procedure. It is as follows. Puta is given after combining suddha kasisa and suddha gandhakam taken in equal parts and thus bhasma is obtained. It is known as kanta Kaseesa. He advocates administering the bhasma in the following way. Equal quantities of kasisa bhasma and Marica churna is mixed and administered in pratahkala in one niska dose with madhu and ghrita. He indicates them in ksaya, gulma, pliharoga sula and mutra roga.

Gairikam (red ochre) : Gairika is of three varieties. Pasana gairikam, swarnagairika and mrt gairikam (rakata gairikam) will have red shine. Gairikam is to be made mardana with appropriate quantity of cows milk for its sodhana or gairika is made Bharjana with goghrta for its sodhana. Gairika used mainly in rakta vikara, rakta pitta (bleeding disorders), hikka, visa and jwara and is chakshushya (good for eyes) and balya (nourishing).

Hingulam (cinnabar) . Hingula originated from mercury and compound of parada and gandhaka which occurs as mineral in the mines. It is associated with other minerals and also made artificially. Chemically it contains

13.8% sulphur and 86.2% mercury.

Hingula sodhana:

Hingula is to be triturated with aja ksira and amla varga drava dravya seven times for sodhana. Hingula is also to be triturate with breast milk or jambira swarasa for its sodhana.

Hinngula marana vidhi: Fine powder of hingula is to be collected in one valla quantity and it is spread on an earthen pot, the one karsa (12 gram) of suddha hingula and two karsa of ardraka swarasa, one masa (1gram) lavanga churna also to be added, then this earthen pot is closed with a small pot made sandhibandhana and heated over mandagni for 3 yama (9hours) . After it got cooled hingula bhasma is to be collected and administered in 1 gunja (125mg) dose with betel leaf. This hingula is nourishing and cures anemia and all types of diseases. Administering of impure Hingula causes skin diseases, impotency and moha (delusion) .

Manahshila (realgar) : It is of 3 varieites. They are shyamangi, Kanavira and dwikhandakya. Contrary to thers, author opines kanaveera is the best. He advocates bhavana with agastya patra swarasa or with ardhraka rasa for 7 times to make manahsila purified. Among these kanavira variety of Manashila is considered as best. Seven bhavanas of manashila with agasthya patra swarasa or ardraka swaraasa to produce sodhita manashila.

Sankha: Very limited information is available about sankha. Simple purification method, such as purification with amlavarga and kanji in dolayantra is advised.

Colour parameters for bhasma:

Parameters set to ensure whether swarna etc bhasma are properly prepared they have put some colours as para meter as follows.

स्वर्णं कपोतकंठाभमारमेवं सदा भवेत् । शुल्बं मयूरकंठाभं तारवंगौ समुज्ज्वलौ ॥५०६॥ कृष्णसर्पनिभं नागं तीक्ष्णं कज्जलसन्निभम् । तदा शुद्धं विजानीयाद् वांति भ्रांति विवर्जितम् ॥५०७॥ एतत्सर्वन्तु जातस्स्यात्पुटानं नसमंभवेत् ।

Swarna should be similar to kapota kanta varna if properly preparaed. The color of tamra bhasma will be similar to colour of mayura kanta. Rajatabhasma vangabasma looks bhasmas prepared basing on the colour. He attributes some colours to dhatus and fixes them as parameter. According to him any deviation from it necessitates to give some more putas to meet the standards. This kind of information at one place is not available in other texts of rasasastra.

The colour of swarna bhasma and pittala bhasma is ujwala. The colour of nagabhasma will be similar to krsna sarpa. The colour of tiksna lauha bhasma will be like kajjali. Properly prepared bhasma wil not cause vanti (vomitings), branti etc adverse reactions. If these adverse reaction occur some more putas are to be given.

Dosage of Bhasma: Another unique feature of this book is the mention of dosage of bhasmas at one place.

Bhasma	**Dosage**
Swarna bhasma	½ valla
Rajata bhasma	½ valla
Tamra Bhasma	½ Valla
Teekshna bhasma	Vallardha to valla

Vangabhasma, pittala basma, naga bhasma ½ valla to valla dose.

सेवनस्य प्रमाणं तु कथयिष्ये हितैषिण: वल्लार्धं कनकं हि सुप्रकथितं रूप्यं च शुल्ब तथा ॥५०६ तीक्ष्णं वंग भुजंगमारभसितं वल्लार्धवल्लोन्मितम् ।
तत्तुल्या शुभपिप्पली निगदिता क्षौद्रं च कर्षान्पितम् ॥५०९ ॥

सेव्यं संपरिहत्य ग्रीष्मशरदौ ताम्रं सुसेव्यं नरै: ।

He prescribes pippali churna and one karsa of honey as general anupana for all bhasmas. Tamra bhasma can be administered in all rtu except grisma and sarat.

Lauhastaka marana vidhi:

तालेन वंगं दरदेन तीक्ष्णं नागेन हेमं शिलया च नागम् ॥ ५१०॥

शुल्बं तथा गंधवरेण नित्यं तारं च माक्षीकवरेण हन्यात् ।

Vangabhasma is to be prepared with haratala. Tikshna lauha bhasma is prepared with Hingula. Swarna bhasma is to be prepared with manahshila and naga. Tamra bhasma is to be prepared with gandhaka. Rajata hasma is to be prepared with Maksika.

Likewise the deleterious effects of saptadhatu due to improper purification given at one place. There are as follows.

Improper purification of swarnabhasma causes fatigue and sweating. Rajata bhasma causes udararoga, agnimanya. If tamra bhasma is not properly prepared vanti, bhranti, Naga and trapu causesanga dosa, gulma and sosa. Asuddha Tiksna lauha bhasma causes sula (pain) . If kanta lauha bhasma not properly prepared then causes krisata (leanness) sphota (boils) . If asuddha pittala is administered then it causes moha.

Upadhatu:

The following seven upadhatu produced by seven dhatus, they are as follows.

स्वर्णजं स्वर्णमाक्षीकं तारजं तारमाक्षिकम् ।। ५१४ ।।

तुत्थं ताम्रभवं ज्ञेयं कंकुष्ठं वंगसंभवम् । रसकोजसदाज्जातो नागात्सिंदूर
संभवः ।।५१५।। लोहाज्जातं लोहकिट्टमेतास्सप्तोपधातवः ।

Swarna makshika is the upadhatu of swarna, Taramakshika is the upadhatu of rajata, tutham derives from tamram, kankusta from vanga, khalkappari from jasada, sindhuram derives from naga, and lohakitta from loha . As per modern alchemy Swarna makshika contains iron (Fe), Copper (Cu) and sulfur.

Substitutes advised in the place of Dhatu

स्वर्णाभावे मृतं ताप्यं ततोपि स्वर्णगैरिकम् ।। ५१६।।

रूप्यादीनामलाभे तु प्रक्षिपेद्विमलादिकम् । ।

When doing formulations in the non-availability of Swarna, It is advised to take Swarna mākṣika or Swarna girika. In non-availability of Rajata, It is advised to take Vimala etc.

Thus in Vaidyacintamani we find all the relevant practical information at one place serves the physicians with a comprehensive outlook on rasasastra which helpin preparing better formulations.

Swarna makshika suddhi: 3 parts of swarnamakshika and 4 parts of saindhavalavana are collected in iron container, then it is filled with jambira swarasa or bijapura nimbu swarasa till the material is immersed and heated to red hot state while stirring with iron rod, then sodhita swarna makshika is obtained.

Hemamakshika Bhasma: Part of swarna makshika mixed with $1/4^{th}$ part of gandhaka and it is triturated with appropriate quantity of eranda thaila and chakrika are prepared. This chakrika are kept in sarava and sandhibandhana is done sarava samputa is kept in Tusa then gajaputa is given. After swanga sitala formed sindhura varna swarmna makshika is collected.

swarnamakshika mixed with eranda thaila, gunja, honey, tankana and triturated then this material is heated to produce swarnamakshika satva.

Swarna Makshika guna: Similar toother rasatantra texts, similar gunas like vrsya (aphrodisiac), rasayanaa (rejuvenative), chakshusya (beneficial to eyes) mentioned. He advocates Triphala churna, Trikatu churna, maricha churna and ghrita as anupana. Advocated to use pure swarnamakshika if not symptoms of indigestion develop. When Tara makshika rubbed over stone it appears shiny and similar to rajata.

Taramakshika: The following information available regarding taramakshika in Vaidyachintamani.

This taramakshika slightly varies with swarna makshika and slightly similar to rajata hence known as Taramakshika.

Describing its sodhana he states that roupya makshika is powdered and given bhavana in karkoti swarasa, meshashringi swarasa and jambeera swarasa for one day each, later it should be exposed to hot sun then sodhita tara makshika is collected.

All the other aspects like guna etc of taramakshika are similar but less effective than swarna makshika and all the adverse reactions mentioned for swarnamakshika are also applicable for taramakshika.

Tuttha (blue vitriol) : The description of tuttha almost similar to that mentioned in yogaratnakara i.e. Tutha is taken equal to the quantity of marjala mala, honey and tankana and given bhavana in amlavarga and cooked along with aswamutra in dolayantra. Badhwashila churna also used for the purpose of sodhana.

We also find description of kshira tutha and maila tutha. Tutha is administered in kandu (itching), worm infestations, and conditions of poison.

Sodhana of Rasaka: Fine powder of rasaka is to be made into pottali with a cloth and it is immersed in naramutra or gomutra and cooked in dolayantra process for seven days to obtain sodhita rasaka. This can be used in all purposes.

Kankusta: Kankusta is tikta and katu in rasa it is given bhavana in shunti kashaya and is repeated for three times. Thus sodhita kankusta is considered as best. It is administered in gulma, udavarta, sula, parad dosha and for wound healing.

Giri sindhura Suddhi: For suddhi of girisindhuram mardana with jambeera drava (nimbu swarasa) and later dried up in the sun. Afterwards given mardana with tandulodaka.

Gauri pashana (white arsenic) : In Vaidyacintamani there is description about gauree pashana, ullipashana, and doddipashana. For purification of gaureepashanam, it is advised to give mardana with Jambeera swarasa and this paste is collected in cloth, made into pottali form and boiled in dola yantra which is filled with lime water for 2 yama (6hours).

Sodhana of Akhupasana: Fine powder of Akhupasana is collected into a cloth and made into pottali form then boiled in dola yantra for 1 day, which is filled with lime water. Sodhana of akhupashana also can be done by boiling in a Dola yantra, which is filled with madhu for 1 yama (3 hours)

Sodhana of rakta pashana: Fine powder of rakta pashana is to be kept in a cloth made into pottali form then is boiled in dola yantra process which is filled with cows urine.

Silajitu:

विदाघे घर्मसंतप्ता धातुसारं धराधरा: । । ५४९ । । निर्यासवत्प्रमुंचन्ति तच्छिलाजतु कीर्तितम् ।

Dhatu sara (exudate from sila) secreting from mountains because of temperature produced by sunlight is called shilajitu. (Mineral pitch).

He mentions about two types of Silajitu i.e gomutra silajitu and karpoora silajitu but did not mention of 5 varities accepted by susruta and charaka etc. These five varieties are hema garbha silajitu, Tara garbha silajitu, amra garbha silajitu, Ayo garbha silajitu, Naga garbha silajitu, Vanga garbha silajitu. Gomutra silajitu is Rasayana, karpura silajitu considered as best.

Sodhana of silajitu: Silajitu is to be immersed in the liquid made up of yavakshara, sarja kshara, amla Drava and guggulu. This material is allowed for drying in sunlight for one day, thereafter swedana to be done in above-mentioned liquid for 1 yama to obtain suddha silajitu.

Sodhana of karpura silajitu: karpura silajitu is to be triturated with mrinala swarasa or utpala swarasa for 1 yama (3 hrs) for its sodhana.

Karpura silajitu is to be triturated with cows milk, triphala kashaya and bhringaraja swarasa simultaneously, then the material is dried in sun light for 1 day for its sodhana. One pala of karpura silajitu is made mardana for seven ghatika with kamala kanda swarasa then this material is to be dried in sunlight.

शुद्धोऽयं गिरितप्रकंदरभवः पांडु प्रमेहज्वरप्लीह
श्लेष्ममरुद्भवाग्निसदनत्वग्दोषशोषपहा ॥५। यक्ष्मोन्मादकशोफशर्करकृमीन्
हच्छूलपित्तापहो । हन्त्याच्चोदरकामिलाश्मरिजराकृच्छ्राणि पामापहा ॥५

Silajitu mainly administered in urinary tract infections, kamala, mutrakrichra etc.

अशुद्धं दाहमूर्छाया भ्रमपित्तास्रशोणितम् । शिलाजतु प्रकुरुते मांद्यमग्नेश्च
विग्रहम्

We also get references of adverse reactions of it such as raktapitta, (bleeding disorders), burning sensation and constipation.

To identify suddha silajitu, shilajitu is put over agni if it becomes into lingakara and dhuma rahita. Shilajitu if put in water should become into tantu (thread) like in appearance, there after dissolved in water and it produces odour similar to gomutra considered to be suddha shilajitu.

Notes:

Shilajit is a natural substance found mainly in the Himalayas, formed for centuries by the gradual decomposition of certain plants by the action of microorganisms. It is a potent and very safe dietary supplement, restoring the energetic balance and potentially able to prevent several diseases. Recent investigations point to an interesting medical application toward the control of cognitive disorders associated with aging, and cognitive stimulation. Thus, fulvic acid, the main active principle, blocks tau self-aggregation, opening an avenue toward the study of Alzheimer's therapy.

Sadharana rasa:

साधारण रसाः केचिद्रसकर्मोपयोगिनः ॥ ५६१ ॥

पूर्वशास्त्रानुसारेण वक्ष्यंते लक्षणादिभिः । कंपिल्लो लवणं गौरीपाषाणो नवसागरम् ॥ ५६

दरदो वह्निजारश्च गिरिसिंदूरमेव च । मृद्दारशृंगं चेत्यष्टौ साधारणरसाः स्मृताः
॥५८

Sadharana rasa which are useful for rasa karya. These are eight types, Kampilla (mallotus philippensis), samudra lavana (sea salt), gauripashana (white arsenic), navasadara (sal ammoniac) hingula, agnijara, girisindhura (red oxide of mercury) and mrddaru srnga (litharge).

Kampilla: Available in saurastra desa in the form of mineral and appears Like brick powder is called kampillaka. It is purgative. Fine powder of kampilla is to be kept in dolayantra, which is filled which haritaki kashaya and swedana is done .The qualities of kampilla are katu, ushna, causes purgation. Relieves from Vrana, kapha, Jantu and krimi. Much description is not available.

Mastaki: Powder of mastaki curna is to be made mardana with jambira (citrus limon) for 1 yama or with human urine for 1 yama (3 hours) for its sodhana.

Author gives description about Sarja Kshara and yava Kshara.

Sarjikasara: sarjika ksara is given mardana with kanji (sour gruel) for two ghatika (6hours) or given mardana with gomutra for its sodhana. Its action mainly is Agni deepana (kindle fire).

Yavaksara (potassium salts) : Fine powder of Yavaksara is to be triturated with tandulodaka (rice water), and then this material is dried in sunlight for 1 ghatika. Yavaksara ia also dipana and kapha vataghna.

Notes:

Ksharas are alkaline substances obtained from the water-soluble ashes of herbal drugs. Several Ksharas have been explained in Ayurveda and Apamarga kshara is one among them. Different opinions exist regarding specifications for the nature of vessels, the proportion of water, time for settling, cloth folding, etc.

Panchalavana:

सैंअथवा छागमूत्रेण पाचितं शुद्धिमाप्नुयात् । निंबूनीरेण सौवर्चं भावयेच्छुद्धिमाप्नुयात् ॥ ५७१ बिडालवणकं तक्रे भावयेच्छुद्धिमाप्नुयात् । लवणं काचकं भाव्यं तिंत्रिणीजल आतपे ॥५७५ समुद्रलवणं लोष्टे तप्तं कुर्यात्त्रियामकम् । सम्यक् शुद्धं भवेद्वैद्यस्त्वौषधेषु प्रयोजयेत् ॥ ५४९

लवणानि क्षालितानि सक्षारेणांभसातपे । शोषितानि विशुध्यन्तीति ज्ञेयं
वैद्यपारगैः धवं कांजिके भाव्यं भवेच्छुद्धिर्घटीद्वये ॥ ५७३

For sodhana of pancha lavana, it is to be made mardana with sour gruel for 2 yama and dried in sun light or saindhavalavan boiled in goat urine to obtain sodhita saindhavalavana.

Sodhita sauvarcalavan is obtained by triturating with Nimbuswarasa and dried in sunlight.

Vidalavana is to be made bhavana with takra and dried in sunlight to obtain sodhita vida lavana.

Kaca lavana is to be made trirurated with tindika jala and dried in sunlight to obtain sodhita kaca lavana.

Samudra lavana is to be heated with over piece of earthen pot for 3 yamas then sodhita samudra lavana is obtained. Thus purified panchalavana are to be added to prepare formulations. All lavana can be cleaned in kashara jala and dried in sun light before adding them in formulations. All lavanas are generally kapha vata roga hara and sula hara and cure kukshiroga.

Trikatu Suddhi:

शुंठीं निस्त्वक्कृतां चाथ शिलाक्षारं विलेपयेत् । निक्षिपेदातपे यामं सम्यक्
शुद्धिर्भवेद्ध्रुवम् ॥ ५८२॥ वैदेहीं चित्रकरसे ह्यातपे भावयेत्तथा । सम्यक्
शुद्धिर्भवेदेतां रसयोगेषु योजयेत् ॥ ५८३॥ मरिचं त्वम्लतक्रेण भावितं
घटिकात्रयम् । लोष्ठे क्षिप्त्वा ततस्तसं शुद्धं भवति निश्चितम् ॥५८४।

The external layer is removed and newly collected lime is to be pasted over the sunthi and dried in sunlight for 1 yama there after sodhita sunthi is collected.

Pipppali is to be immersed in chitramula kashaya for 2 ghatika and then dried in sunlight to obtain sodhita pippali.

Marica is to be triturated in amla takra for three ghatika and roasted in earthen pot in order to obtain sodhita marica. Thus sodhita trikatu used in the preparation of rasaoushadhi. There is mention of gaja pippali bhavana with goat urine to obtain sodhita gajapippali.

Sodhana of ahiphena: Ahiphena (papaver somniferum) is to be placed over the leaves of gajakarna patra and pottali is made and kept in dola yantra which is filled with cows milk and boiled for 1 yama 3hours, thereafter mineral is taken out and dried.

Sodhana of hingu (ramatha) :

Hingu is to be triturated with kamala patra (nelumbo lucefera) swarasa for 1 yama therafter material is dried in sun light and sodhita hingu is obtained. And used in the preparation of rasayoga.

Sodhana 2 types of Jiraka:

The two varieties of jiraka i.e sweta jiraka and Krishna jiraka are to be immersed in kanji (sour gruel) for 2 yama There after this material is taken out and slightly roasted and sodhita jiraka is obtained.

Sodhana of eranda bija and danti bija:

Visamusti bija is to be boiled in tanduliya mula (Amarantus spinosus)

(Chaulayi vegitable amaranthus campstria) swarasa for three ghatika thereafter sodhita visamusti is obtained.

Sodhana of nepala bija (jaipala bija):

Thin external ayer of jaipala bija (croton tiglium) is to be removed and it should be cooked in kumara swarasa gudodaka (jiggery mixed with water), cow'milk, cow'ghee separately thereafter sodhita jaipala bija is obtained.

Vasanabhi:

The synonym is visham. Visham (Vatsanabhi) should be cut into pieces and tied in a cloth bolus (pottali) and kept in a pot, gomutra poured in to the pot in order that the bolus gets submerged. This pot is kept in the sun for 3 days. Everyday Cow's urine has to be replaced with the new. On the fourth day Vatsanabhi is taken out and dried up in sunlight and made into powder to be used in medicines.

RASA KARPOORA: We get vivid description about rasakarpoora. Rasabhasma when undergoes murcha and attains urdhwapatana (Upward distillation) known as Rasakarpoora. The dose given is gunja pramana. Since it cures many diseases it is known as Mahakarpoora. It is condered as Rasabheda. It is administerd either in valla pramana or ½ valla pramana. It is given along with old jaggery or depending on the clinical condition suitable anupana is selected and administered. Milk and rice are advised as pathyam. It is mainly used in Phirangaroga (syphilis), all types of kusta and vrana. It is also been said to improve the virility, digestion and also complexion as gold.

Navratna:

We get information about vajra (diamond), vidruma (pravala), mukta (pearl), marakata (emerald), vaidhurya (cat's eye), gomeda, manikya (ruby), hrinila (sapphire), pusparaga (topaz) which are considered as navaratna. Description of uparatna also available.

Author recommends sodhana for all types of ratna because asuddha ratna produces different adverse reactions. Manikya with amla dravya, mukta with jayanti swarasa, pravala with ksira varga, tarksya with godugdha, pusparaga with saindhavalavana and kulatha kwatha, vajra with tanduliyakaswarasa, nilam with nili swarasa, gomedha with gorochana jala, vaidurya with triphalakashaya swedana is to be done with dolayantra process for their sodhana.

Maranam: Marana is not recommended for costlier ratna, If it is does so, the person attains gaurava pataka. He advocates sodhana for less costlier ratnas possessing similar gunas. Mardana in manasila, gandhakam, talakam and kuchala Drava, and subjecting it to 8 putas are required to make bhasma. Marana could be done for all such ratnas except vajra. He denounces the use of asuddharatna since they cause visphota (boils), tapa (heat sensation), bhrama, daurbalya (weakness) and veeryanasa. **Notes:** *Initially the Metals & Minerals must undergo for Purification with prescribed herbal juice or with decoction for a stipulated time. Then it should be treated with appropriate amount of fire. This process has to be repeated till we get appropriate Bhasma lakshana. This process is known as Marana.*

Vajra:

Sodhana of vajra: vajra is to be cooked in dola yantra with kulatha kwatha or kodrava kwatha. Then vajra material is taken out and kept in vyaghri khanda, then covered with mud and cloth, thereafter puta is given continuously for 1 day and night. Self cooling the material is taken out cleaned by spraying wth horse urine or snuhi ksira for sodhana of vajra. Vajra should be collected in the auspicious day and inserted in vyaghrimula and covered with buffalo dung, then it is kept in cowdung cakes and puta is given for 4 yama in the night, after that vajra is collected and immersed in horse urine. This puta is repeated for seven times to obtain sodhita vajra.

Sodhana and marana of Vajra:

त्रिः सप्तकृत्वः संप्तसं खरमूत्रेण शुध्यति । मत्कुणैस्तालकं पिष्ट्वा तद्गोले कुलिशं क्षिपेत् ॥ ६१ प्रध्यातं वाजिमूत्रेण सिक्तं पूर्वं क्रमेण वै । भस्मीभवति तद्व्रजं शंखशीतांशु पांडुरम् ॥ ६२

Nirvapana (process of reducing red hot elements in liquid media) of vajra is to be done in khara mutra and this procedure is to be repeated for 21 times in order to obtain the suddha vajra.

Haratala is to be triturated with khatmal and this material is made into circular mass. Then vajra is to be inserted in to that circular mass. Thereafter this total mass is kept in the andha musa then sandhibandhana is to be made and gajaputa is given. Like this, after completing seven puta vajrabhasma gets prepared.

Vajra bhasma is very efficacious hence is administered with different anupana depending on the disease.

कुष्ठे खादिरकं शृतंपवनयुग्रक्ते समध्वाकम् । कासश्वासबलासकेषु सकणात्वग्वासकृष्णद्रवम् ॥ ६२ पित्ते दाहयुते सितां ज्वरगदे च्छिन्ना जलं तिक्तकम् । वज्रे मारित शुक्लभस्मनि भिषक् संयोज्य दद्यात्सदा

Vajra bhasma administered with Khadira Kashaya in Kustu.

Vajra bhasma administered with Ardhraka Swarasa, Honey in Vatavyadhi.

Vajra bhasma administered with Vasa Kashayam in Vatarakta.

Vajrabhasma Qualities: It inreases the longevity and strength makes one good looking and ensures comfort to the body. Thus he has described the good effects in general. And also cautions that asuddha vajra bhasma causes kusta, parsva vedana, pandu, tapa jadatva etc.

Pravala (corals): A very little description is given for pravala. We find only one suddhi procedure i.e. bhavana with Jambeera Swarasa for one prahara 3hrs, later it is washed with warm water.

To prepare bhasma bhavana is given in arka ksira for 3 days, then pellets are prepared, later gajaputa is given to obtain pravala bhasma.

Pravala cures Raktapitta, Raktatisara, pradara and Raktashulaghnam.

Raktasulaghnam a typical term used not mentioned in any other text. Its suddhi procedure is simple and easily available. Even today the general practitioners of medicine use pravala mainly to control bleeding.

Mukta (pearl) : Mauktikam should be done sodhana with amlavarga, kanjika, Jambeeraswarasa or gomutra and again swedana is to be done with godugdha to obtain suddha mukta.

Second method:

1) Kundalee swarasa or Tintrinidrava tamarindus indica for 3 days to obtain suddha mukta.

to get bhasma of mukta, it is given bhavana with sweta brihatiphala swarasa, then pellets are prepared and dried. These pelettes are processed in bhuputa inorder to obtain mukta bhasma. Mukta bhasma is sita virya (cooling property) and madhura rasa hence mainly used in pitta roga and daha and also as styptic.

Pushparagam: Author advocates suddhi of puspharagam either with goats urine or pashanabhedhi swarasa and then pelletes are prepared and given Viswakarma puta to prepare bhasma.

Pushparaga is pustikaram (nourishing), slesmalam, guru (heavy) and seetalam (cooling).

No specific disease indication is given. He deleted much of the information related to pushparagam like mythological origin, varieties, and qualities when compared to ther texts.

Marakata (emerald): Marakata is kept inside of vidarikanda by chiselling it. Later it is given kukkuta puta for making shodhana of it. He advocates kantakari swarasa bhavana, pashanabhedhi swarasa for mardana and later chakrika are prepared and subjected to one gajaputa.

Qualities of Marakata: Clear, delighting, laghu, causes constipation and alleviates tridosha.

Vaidhurya (cats eye): Author advises bhavana of vaidhurya with horse urine for one day and later in kushmanda Swarasa for one day to obtain suddha vaidhurya.

For making bhasma he advocates bhavana with shilabhedhi rasa (pashanabheda swarasa) later chakrikas are prepared and dried then heated in viswakarma puta (goldsmiths funnel), therafter the material collected into vajra musa and, sandhibandhana is done and subjected to gajaputam to obtain vaidhurya bhasma.

He opines that in qualities it is similar to Vajra and is capable of curing all diseases.

Gomedhika (hessonite, cinnamon stone) : Author advocates simple suddhi procedures for gomedhika too. This is as follows, 3 days bhavana in horse urine, later it is to be soaked in vidarikanda swarasa to obtain suddha gomedika.. He advocates bhavana with Krishna dattura swarasa for 3 days and chakrika are to be prepared, then viswakarma puta is to be given in order to obtain gomedaka bhsma. It is kapha hara, digestant and imparts strength. But he did not give any disease indication for it.

Manikya (ruby) : Author advocates bhavana of manikya in horse urine for 3 days then it is to be exposed to sun rays and later washed with hot water to obtain suddha manikya . Bhavana of suddha manikya is done with arka ksira and then cakrika are to be prepared and dried. These chakrikas are kept in sarava samputa, thereafter three putas are given in order to obtain manikya bhasma. It is Nourishing, beneficial increasing the life span. And improves complexion.

Nilam (sapphire) : For purification of neela it is given bahvana in urine of donkey for one day and exposed to hot sun to obtain suddha Nilamani. It is triturated with lakshmana patra swarasa for three yama (9hrs) and chakrika are made and dried, there after viswakarma puta is given in order to obtain Nila bhasma.

The qualities are seeta, guru, snigdha, and madhura and pitta nasana. The description of ratnas and uparatnas have been minimized in the text and also advised very simple suddhi and bhasma procedures, probably due to their limitation in clinical efficacy.

Vaikranta (tourmaline) : Vaikranta is of eight kinds i.e sweta, rakta, pita, nila, paravataprabha, syama, krisna karpura varna . Any one variety among nila, sweta and lohita Varna variety of vaikranta is to be processed on the lines of vajra sodhana vidhi. In order to obtain suddha vaikranta (tourmaline) nirvapana of vaikranta is to be done in asva mutra for 21 times. Indravaruni panchanga is to be triturated and made into golaka form suddha vaikranta is to be immersed into that golaka and externally covered with cloth and mud and dried thereafter seven puta is to be given to obtain bhasma. We also get description about vaikranta driti (drava) and also of vaikranta satvapatana (One method of extraction of essence from mineral ores) .

Vaikranta improves life span and is digestant, nourishing cures all diseases and eliminates poison.

Sodhana: Vaikranta becomes purified if it is subjected to boiling for 3 days in the following liquids containing ksharas (alkalies), lavanas (salts) . The liquids are amla dravas (acidic liquids), mutras (urines) and the decoctions of mulatha, rambha or kodrava .It is also purified by subjecting it to svedana (boiling) in kulatha kwatha.

YANTRA PRAKARANAM

Rasashastra deals with metallic, mineral and poisonous drugs. These drugs are pharmaceutically processed and rendered fit for internal administration. For the various processing of rasa uparasadi dhatus and for the preparation of medicines, specific apparatuses called 'Yantras' are needed.

Author of vaidyachintamani allotted separate chapter for yantra prakarana.

Some of the commonly using yantras mentioned in Vaidya chintamani are as follows

Vidhyadhara yantra:

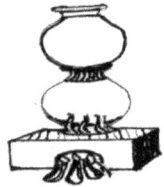

A large size container is taken and parada is kept in that and another container is put over that and sandhibandhana is done. The upper container should be filled with water, lower container is kept over fire and heated for five prahara (3 hours) . After swanga shitala, sandhibandhana is removed and parada collected which is adhered to the lower surface of upper container with brush and this is called vidhayadhara yantra .

Tanka Yantra:

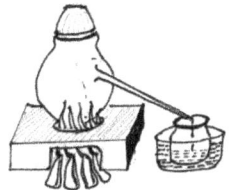

A earthen pot is taken and pierced (hole) at its neck region so as to place a wooden tube. Another pot placed over the mouth of first pot having the same size of the mouth. Later it is sealed with mud and cloth (both earthen pots and hole where wooden bamboo pierced), another end of bamboo pipe should be in a glass container, to collect distilled essence coming out as drops. The earthen is kept over furnace and contents are boiled. Because of distillation process the medicament is collected into glass container. This yantra is known as tankana yantra.

Valuka yantra :

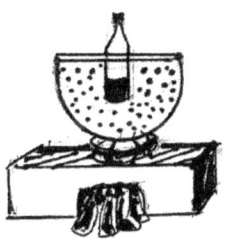

भांडे वितस्ति गंभीरे मध्ये निहितकूपिके । कूपिकाकंठ पर्यंतं वालुकाभिश्च पूरयेत् ॥ ६ ॥ भेषजं कूपिकासंस्थं वह्निना पाचयेत्ततः । वालुकायंत्रमेतद्धि यंत्रतंत्रबुधैः स्मृतम् ॥७॥

Bhanda which is having one vitasti depth (A vitasti (Sanskrit: वितस्ति, vitasti) is an ancient Indian unit of length approximating to 21 centimeters.) and width is to be taken and a vertical glass bottle which is pasted with cloth and mud further filled with medicinal ingredients (kajjali etc) is kept in the central portion of the container then the container should be filled with sand to the level of neck of the bottle. Thereafter this container is kept over the fire and heated as per the procedure then this is called valukayantra.

Garbha Yantra:

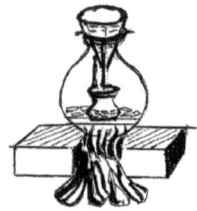

One big bhanda is taken and bricks are kept in side the bhanda, a small container equal to the size of ghatika is filled with cold water and kept over big container vertically underneath to this container a glass bottle should be hanged, by keeping over the brick and sandhibandhana is done in between the joint of big container and the container having the shape of ghatika (bell) .Fire is given in the lower container and when the water of the container becomes hot, then it should be changed.Suandhita taila or arka will be collected in glass container .This is called garbha yantra, it is used extract sugandhita taila and arka etc.

Kacchapa yantra:

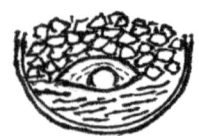

A wide vessel is taken and filled with mrttika (soil), in its central portion parada and bida is placed, then covered with a small earthen container. The junction of small earthen container and mrttika is sealed then coal made up of wood is to be put over the yantra, then fire is given. This kacchapa yantra used for gandhaka jarana with parada.

Jala Yantra:

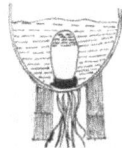

Water in upper portion, fire source will be down portion and parada and gandhaka is to be plaed in between. This jala yantra is considered best yantra .By using this yantra swarna etc.satva and gandhaka etc., jarana will be prepared. To make this yantra one big iron container is to be taken Parada, swarna, gandhaka etc are to be collected in an iron musa and it is closed with a lid.Then the external surface of this musa is to be pasted with loha churna mixed with ajarakta (goat blood) and dried.Paste made with mixture of old brick powder, guda triturated with babbula kwatha and this paste is applied over the loha musa (crucible) khadiya lavana loha kitta churna are to be triturated with buffalo milk and this paste is to be applied over the musa in order to avoid the leakage of parada. Then this musa is to be given fire from underneath surface of the container.

Gauree Yantra:

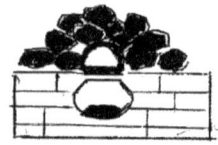

Gauri yantra used for jarana process. A brick having eight angula length and width is ito be taken in its central place of the brick a pit is made like musa and lime is to be pasted in the pit to make the surface smooth.Then roupya, swarna etc., sattva are taken and filled in pit (musa made in the brick) . Underneath to this sattva and above the sattva roupya, swarna etc $1/4^{th}$ quantity to this sattva of gandhaka is covered. Then they are covered by small earthen pot, thereafter sandhana is done in the junction of brick and small earthen pot.Then this total instrument covered with cow dung cakes equal to the size of the foot of the horse. And laghu puta is given and this is named as gauri yantra.

Notes :

Jarana involves conversion of Parad like elements into their natural form without using Galena process. Properties of Parada get enhanced when it treated with Gandhaka. Murchhana involves conversion of mercury into compatible, for this purpose sometimes sulphur may be employed for treating mercury.

Vajramusa:

वर्तुला गोस्तनाकारा वज्रमूषा प्रकीर्तिता ॥ २९ ॥ ।

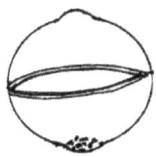

Two parts of ash produced by tusa (husk), one part of valmika mrittika, one part f loha kitta, one part of sweta pasana churna, little quantity of human hair together are collected and mixed with appropriate quantity of aja dugdha then boiled till contents becomes into concentrated form.Then mardana of these for two yama (6hours) is to be done till the material becomes soft in consistency. There after this material moulded to musa similar to the shape of circular, Gostana (breast) . Like this two musa are to be prepared. And the mouth of the parada containing is to be joined with the mouth of another Musa and sandhibandhana is to be done This vajra musa is used for parada marana.

Bhudhara yantra:

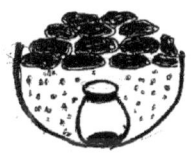

Parada is taken in a musa and its mouth is sealed with cloth and soil, there after one big container with wide opening is to be taken, half of its volume is filled with sand within the sand musa is placed, over that sand cow dung cakes are placed and fired.This instrument is called bhudhara yantra.

Kosti Yantra:

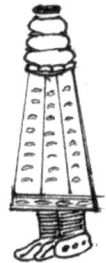

One hasta pramana bamboo stick tube is to be taken, at the one end of the stick cloth is to be tied, the another end at the length eight angula is to be made bent, this bent end is introduced into the ground at the tip of this and cool is filled and this cool is fired compressing cloth bag and by blowing air this is called kosti yantra.

Notes: *In order to extract the satwa (metallic part) from the ores aswell as to purify it, kostis (furnace stove) of different size and shape are necessary.*

Dola yantra:

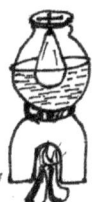

In a bhurjapatra (betula utilis) parada along with other medicinal substances is to be collected into it and tied, thereafter it is to be placed over the three times folded cloth then tied tightly with a thread and in the central part of the bamboo stick, thereafter this bamboo stick should be kept over the mouth of the earthen pot and pottali should be hanged in an earthen pot (which is already filled with medicinal liquids like kanji etc.) this earthen pot should be kept over the kosti and the contents are cooked as per the time prescribed for the swedana process.this is called Dola yantra .

Tula yantra:

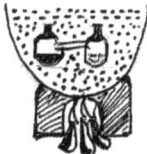

2 musas are to be prepared similar to the shape of the brinjal. Among these 2 musas one musa should be filled with suddha parada and another musa should be filled with suddha gandhaka. Both the musas are connected with a pipe and sandhi badhana is made. Then this which are appearing like tula is to be placed in valuka yantra and this valuka antra is heated over agni. Heat should be given underneath the gandhaka containing Musa. This Tula yantra is oftenly used to make satwajarana from haratala, gandhaka etc.

Patala yantra:

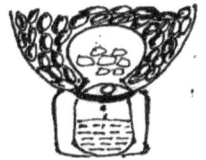

A pit about one hasta depth is to be made in ground. At the bottom of pit one container with wide mouth should be kept.In one sarava (earthen pot) medicinal drug is to be taken and its mouth should be packed with fine mesh in order to get filter the oil/dravaka.The mouth of saravika inverted position should be placed on the bottom of another big earthen container which is having a hole at its bottom.Then the big earthern container along with sarava should be placed over the wide mouthed container facing the hole of big earthern container on the mouth of wide mouthed container which is present in the pit sandhibandhana is to done at the joint place between the big earthern container the mouth of wide mouthed container.then rest of the surrounding area movements of bhanda. Then cowdung cakes are placed over the big earthgern container. Thereafter fire is given. With this heat, the drugs inside the sarava start exuding gradually through mesh and hole. The oil will trickle down to the wide mouthed container kept in the pit. After swanga sital this taila is to be collected carefully and this yantra is called as patal yantra and it was told by god sambhu by himself.

Tejo yantra:

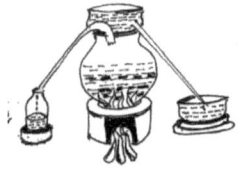

One big bhanda is taken and half of its volume is to be filled with arka dravya and water. Above the bhanda, a small container filled with cold water is to be kept and the joint to be sealed. This small container is fixed with a pipe, the other end of the pipe is kept in another container, which is kept on the ground for collecting hot water from the upper container. This small container is fixed with one more pipe, one end of this pipe should be opened in he bottom of the small container to collect the condensed arka and the end of the pipe is kept in a glass bottle to collect the arka drop by drop.This tejo yantra is basically used for distillation process and this also called lambika yantra .

Puta:

Notes:

Puta is the process in which the degree of heat, which is necessary for the incineration of rasa, maharasa, uparasa or metals, is understood.It is seen that the degree of heat is neither less, nor more than necessary, in this process. Puta helps in converting the metals, minerals into bhasma.thus they become minute and also potentiated to get absorbed in to the body and get digested when once administered.

To get into bhasma form different types of metals, minerals gems and jewels need application of different amount of heat. Hence, They are processed in a specially designed fire place called puta.Depending upon the heat requirement some of them are arranged in pits of different sizes drugs in the earth and some others are done over the ground .Cow dung cakes generally used as fuel. Metal etc., are kept inside two earthen plates put face to face and the joint sealed with the help seven layers mud smeared cloth. Before cooking, this sealed container is well dried . The main purpose of the puta is to cook material with the required quantity of heat constantly for a sufficient period.Once ignited all the cow dung should be allowed to burn .When the fire is over and the fire place cooled down, the container should be removed. The layers of mud smeared cloth which were used for sealing the joint should then be scrapped into two plates separated to remove the metal etc., inside for further processing.

The following are the important putas mentioned in vaidyacintamani.

Mahaputa: One pit is made in the depth of two hastha and cow dung cakes are filled into the half portion of this pit.then saravasamputa is kept over it. Cow dung cakes are filled till the level of ground surface. Then cow dungs are fired, after swanga sitala sarava samputa is taken out, this is called mahaputa.

Gajaputa :

घनमानवशात् सार्धहस्ते चैव तु गर्तके ॥ ५३ ॥

पूर्ववद्वितरेच्चाग्निस्तत्पुटं गजसंज्ञितम् । माहिषं वेत्ति संज्ञेयं सूरिभिः समुदाहृतम् ॥५४॥

Pit is made in the depth of one and half hasta then sarava samputa is kept and over that cow dung cakes are filled till the level of ground surface.then cow dungs cakes are fired, after swanga sitala, sarava samputa is taken out This is known as gajaputa or mahisa puta as per the great scholars of rasasastra.

Varaha puta :

अरत्निमात्रे गर्ते यद्दीयते पूर्ववत्पुटम् । करीषाग्नौ तु तत्प्रोक्तं पुटं वाराहसंज्ञितम्
॥ ५५ ॥ A squire pit having a depth of one aratni is prepared, cow dung cakes are filled insimilar to gajaputa, then the puta is to given fire .This puta is called as varahaputa.

Kukkuta puta:

वितस्तिमात्रगर्ते यत्पुट्यते तत्तु कौक्कुटम् ।

A squire pit having a depth one vitasti is prepared, filled with cow dung cakes then puta is to be given and this puta is called as kukkutaputa.

Notes: *Kukkuta is cock and the puta is similar to it in size is known as kukkutaputa.*

Kapota puta :

Prepare a squire of having a depth of one vitasti, fill with seven or eight cow dung cakes then puta is to be given, and this puta is called as kapotaputa.

Gobara puta:

As the name indicates, gobara curna (cow dung powder) is used in this puta as fuel instead of upala (cowdung cakes) .Drug containing sarava samputa is to be kept in between cowdung powder, thereafter fire is given and it is called gobaraputa. It is also small puta and recommended for preparing rasa bhasma.

Kumbha puta:

A big earthen pot is taken and at its bottom forty holes having the size of one angula are made. Half quantity of this earthen pot is to be filled with coal, over this medicinal drug is to be kept. Then this container is covered with an earthen plate and sandhibandhana is to be done, therafter dried under caya sushka (cooling under the shade of the sun) procedure. Then this big earthen pot containing holes is to be kept over the cullika (furnace) and heated continuously for three days by fecilitating the entry of fire through holes into the coal. After swanga sitala the processed medicine is to be collected. This is called kumbha puta according to scholars.

MANA PRAKARANAM (WEIGHTS AND MEASUREMENTS)

Ayurveda has its own system of measurement, under the title "Mana Paribhasha". The word mana means to measure. Mana is nothing but a system of measurement, which includes height, weight, volume, length, capacity etc. In vaidya intamani we find followinng information about weights and measurements.

Measurement of Prashta

Fluid items like narikelajala, gomutra etc., 32 pala (pala is 48 grams) considered as prastha.

Aushadhi usedfor extracting swarasa and making kalka 16 pala are considered prastha.

For Taila madhu, ghrta 20 pala is considered as prastha.

For milk 30 pala, dahi 25pala, guda 18 pala, laksa 21 pala are considered as pastha.

Magadha prastha:

प्रस्थं तु षोडशपलं द्रव्ये क्वाथे रसे तथा । क्षौद्रे सर्पिषि तैले च प्रस्थं त्रिंशत्पलं भवेत् ॥३॥

इत्यागमेन द्वैगुण्यं निरामातु द्रव्स्य च ।

Accordinng to magadhamana, aushadhi used for extracting swarasa and making kwatha, 16 palaas considered as prastha. Taila, madhu, ghrta 30 pala are considered as prastha. In a recipe if wet drugs are added in double the quantity, therapeutically they will be as effective as the dry drugs.

Prastha according to bhoja mana is payasa, gommutra, narikela jala 32 pala are prastha.

Mula, twak kasta, patra, phala, lavana, mrittika loha cowdung 16 pala is prastha.

Aushadi used for extracting swarasa, taila, madhu, ghrta dugdha 20 pala is prastha.

Dadhi 25 pala is prastha.

Guda 17 pala is considered as prastha and it is equal to ten niska.

For measuring following items i.e karpoora, kumkuma, kasturi, sarkara, snuhi ksira, vamanadravya, niruha vasti dravya, rakta mokshana dravya 13 ½ pala are considered as prastha.

According to magadhamana container, which is having following measurementsi.e width of 6 angula and length of 12 angula, is considered to measure the volume of 1 prastha.

Sadharana tulamana: According to Aurabhra maharsi 2 gunja is 1 masa, 20 masa is 1 niska and 10 niskas are 1 pala. Hundred pala makes 1 tula.

Description of various measurements: When a beam of a sun rays comes to dark room through a hole present in the roof of the room, the suspended particles seen in this beam of light rays called one raja kana trasarenu or vamsi. Thirty paramanu constitute one trasarenu or vamsi.

Six vamsi makes 1 marici; Six marici makes one rajika. 8 sarsapa makes 1 yava.

4 yava makes 1 gunja.

6 gunja makes 1 masa which is synonymous with hema and dhanyaka.

4 masa makes 1 sana, it is synonymous with dharana and tanka

2 tankas constitute 1 kola its synonymous with ksudramo, vataka and dranksana.

2 kola constitute 1 karsa synonymous with panimanika, aksa, picu, panitala, kincipani

2 karsa constitute 1 ardhapala and its synonymous with sukti and astamika.

2 sukti constitute 1 pala.

2 pala constitute prasriti or prastra.

2 prasritis constitute 1 anjali.

2 kudava constitute 1 manika.

2 sarava constitute 1 prastha.

4 prastha constitute 1 adhaka .

4 adhaka constitute 1 drona.

2 drona constitute 1 surpa.

2 surpa constitute 1 droni.

4 droni constitute 1 khari.

2 thousand pala constitute 1 bhara.

100 pala constitute 1 Tula.

PARIBHASA PARAKARANAM

Referring about kandasara (root or rhizomes) author mentions that like vidari haridra, musta, satavari, rasna sariba, varahi vanasurana aswagandha are to be used in formulations.

Speaking about mulasara (root) author mentions about drugs like brihati, kantakari, saliparni, punarnava sarapunkha lamajjaka, gokshura, its roots should be used in formulations.

Referring to mulatwak sara (root bark) like trivrit, karavira, chitraka and nili its mulatwak sara to be used in formulations.

Darutwak sara: Author advocates the bark stem belonging to lodhra, daruharidra, jambu, dalchini, karanja, to be used in formulations.

Sara sara : Heart wood of madhuka, candana, rohini, devadaru, khadira nimba are called sara to be used in formulations.

Patra sara: Leaves of bhringarajam bhumymalaki, patola, karavellaka, palasa, agnimantha, tulasi, lakshmana, brahmi are called patrasara.

Puspa sara: Flowers of campa, ketaki, asoka, yuthika, shigru utpala dhataki utpala and japa are called puspasara.

Phala sara: Fruits of Draksa, dadima, kharjura, panasa, amra, lakuca, paravata badara kapitha, valliphala are called phala sara.

Bija Sara:

Raktasali, mudga, eranda bija, simbidhanya jyotishmati, kuberaksha, karanja, jatiphala, mayuraka, sigru, pippali, marica, jiraka haritaki, amalaki, vibhitaki vidanga are called bijasara and they are used for the treatment of diseases.

Ksara sara: ksara made up of trivrit, citraka, snuhi putikaranja patala, paribhadra, mundi, ajagandha arjuna, devadaru, sigru bhastrna are called ksara sara.

Ksira sara: ksira obtained from Tilvaka, arka, mahavriksa snuhi, varakanyaka are called ksira sara.

Niryasa sara: the niryasa of stauneya, sarjarasa, srivasa, devadhupa, turuska, palasa, salmali, guggulu, aragwadha, nimba, khadira, bilva, ahiphena are called Niryasa sara.

Sarvanga sara: Whole parts of bhringaraja, patola, pippalimula, bhunimba, durva, prasarini parpata are called sarvanga sara.

Ardra dravya: vasa, kutaja, kushmanda, amrta, tagara, eranda lasuna kharjura, kamalanala, modaki are all should be used in wet form.

Nistavagausadha (materials should be used after removing their external cover like sunti, guduchi, abhiru, lasuna, satavari etc.

Alabdapatinidhi dravya:

In the preparation of a formulation if the part of a plant not specified then the root of the plant is to be used. Because root of the plant considered most potential part of the plant. If root is not present in a particular plant, in such condtions, similar to root rhizome etc., may be taken.

Pratinidhi dravya: If draksa is not available in its place kharjura, marica in place of pippali, sunthi in place of rasna, jatamansi in place of yastimadhu, kantakari in place of bharangi etc can be used.

Notes:

The Abhava Pratinidhi Dravya or herbal substitutes means the Dravya having similar pharmacological activities as like that of original Dravya but may not have similar appearance. The concept of Pratinidhi Dravya is not new, many Pratinidhi dravyas (substitutes) are mentioned in Ayurvedic texts, especially in Bhavaprakasha, Yogaratnakar, Bhaishajya ratnavalli etc. The principle to select Pratinidhi dravyas is based upon Rasa (Taste), Guna (Property), Virya (Potency), Vipaka (effects on digestion) and most significant factor Karma (Action) . The main drug in a formulation should not be substituted; only accessory drugs can be substituted.

Pratinidhi dravya for ashtavarga also been given. Eg ksirakakoli if not available satavari is to be taken. If jivaka is not available kolaparni is to be taken.

We get description of group of drugs having similar functions given collective name. They are as follows.

Panchakola: Pippali, pippalimula, cavya, citraka, sunthi known as panchakola is given.

Dasamula: Bilva, gambhari, tarkari, pathala, syonaka salaparni, prisniparni, kantakari, brihati and gokshura are mentioned as dasamula.

Maha panchamula: bilva, agnimantha, syonaka, gambhari, pathala are collectively called mahapanchamula.

Madyapanchamula: Bala, punarnava, eranda, masaparni, and mudgaparni are collectively called as madyapanchamula.

Kanista panchamula: salaprni, prisniparni, brihati, kantakari, gokshura are collectively called kanista pancamula.

Jivanakya panchamula: Abhiru, vira, jivanti, jivaka, rsabhaka are collectively called as jivanakhya panchamula.

Trnapanchamula: darbha, kas, iksu, sali, sara are trna panchamula.

Amlapanchaka: Bijapura, jambira, Naranga, amlavetasa, cinca are collectively called amlapanchaka.

Pancanga: Tvak, patra, phala, mula, puspa are pancanga.

Panchalavana: Sauvarcala, bida, saindhava, kaca samudralavana are pancalavana.

Pancaksara: Palasa kshara, Muskakakshara, yavakshara sarjakshara, tilakshara are known as pacakshara.

Astaksara: palasa, sigru, apamarga, varuna, arka, yavakshara, sarjika kshara tankana are collectively called as astakshara.

Ksharasatka: tilakshara, langali, vaca, apamarga, sigru, kutaja, muskaka are collectively called as ksarasatka.

Trikshara: sarjikakshara, yavakshara, tankana are collectively called as trikshara

Panca sugandhani: Kasturi, kumkuma, karpura, chandana, gorochana are collectively called as pancha sugandha and these are used as odorant agents and in medicinal preparation.

Pancha pallava: Udumbara, vata aswattha, plaksha, amra are panchapallava.

Panchavalkala: Vata, udumbara, aswtha, plksha, pilu are pancha valkalaUdumbara, vata plaksha, pilu are pancha valkala.

Trijataka-chaturjataka: Ela, lavanga tejapatra, are trjataka anf if nagakesara is added it is known as chaturjataka.

Triphala: Fruit pulp of Haritaki, amalaki and vibhitaki are triphala.

Trikatu: Pippali.marica, sunthi are collectively called as trikatu.,

Chaturbhadra: Sunthi, ativisa, musta, guduchi are collectively called as Caturbhadra.

Lavanatraya: Saindhava lavana, sauvarcala lavana, vidalavana are called lavana traya.

AMAZING PRESCRIPTIONS, METHODS OF PREPARATIONS AND ADMINISTERING METHODS

Administering of medicines with just one or two drugs in a wide range of clinical conditions shows his enormous knowledge in pharmacology and clinical experience aswell. He advocated most of the time ekamulika prayoga (single drugs) or simple formulations involving two or three drugs. Above all, his confidence of indicating a particular yoga as a cure to one particular disease is highly rewarding. It is evident by the fact that throught his book vaidyachintamani with exception of very few almost all yogas single disease indication is mentioned. This shows his excellent command on drugs, and in many instances he has administered similar medicine in number of diseases with mere change of anupana or adding up of churnas relevant to respective diseases.

The following are some of the examples:

1) Sweta erandamula added with saindhavalavam to relieve Vata shula (shula prakaranam) .

2) Mandara mulika churnam added with milk relieves one from Vata shula.

3) Karanja Churnam added with souvarchala lavana to relieve vata shula.

4) Usheeram Pippalee mulam added more ghee to relieve hridaya shula.

5) Sankhabhasma with hot water relieves Pankthishula.

6) Riper beejapura swarasa with saindhaiva lavanam relieves severe heart pain.

7) Varuna kashayam indicated in sannipata gulma, and hridaya shula

8) Amalaki phalam macerated and taken along with milk or Badari patra kalka to relieve from swarabhedam.

9) Maricha churnam added with ghee indicated in vataja Swarabheda.

10) Palasa Satapusha Kwatham cures all prameha.

11) Churna of Ela along with takra or madya cures mutrakrichra

12) Rishabhaka mula Kashayam indicated in mutraghatam.

13) Nagabala mulam along with milk indicated in hridroga, swasa, and kasa.

14) Harina sringa bhasma with ghee relieves hridayashula.

15) Suska gambharika phala kalkam along with milk cures seta pittam

16) Abhaya kalkam with gomutram cures Sleepadam

17) Vriddhadaru churnam gomutram cures sleepada

18) Taka twacha kalka indicated in Vata Vrana.

19) Kuberaksha kalka indicated to relieve all types of pains.

20) Churna of purified vishamusti beeja taken 6 or 7or 8 (seeds) added with sarkara (misri) relieves from raktarsa (bleeding piles) mahameha, twak dosha and krimi.

Likewise we get number of examples describing single drug or with two drugs author confidently administered in treating diseases. But he did not explains how these medicines act on dosa, or in what stage of a diseae.

The following are the peculiarities observed in the preparation of medicines.

While describing the preparation Raja mriganka rasa. We see the peculiar style of advising to add up specific number of drugs like 10 pippali, 19 maricha is interesting

Likewise in the preparation of Hararudraras (Kshaya Prakaranam) we observe peculiar pattern of drug mixing i.e. increasing in quantity i.e. Teekshna bhasma 1 part, Tamra bhasma 2 parts, nagabhasma 3 parts, rajata bhasma 4 parts, swarnabhasma 5 parts, sodhita rasam 6 parts. In many of the roushadhas preparation we find the adding up of maricha in equal quantity of other drugs used in a given yoga

We oberve many a time that the following such as maricha, gandhaka, sarkara, pippalee churna taken in equal quantity to the total quantity of the other drugs used in a given yoga .Selection of such churna probably aimed at potentiating the action of the formulation in the direction of desired clinical action. The following are some of the examples.

Kumudeswararas: We observe equal quantity of manishila 1/4, loha bhasma added half to the quantity of all ingredients.

In the making of Navaratna raja mriganka rasa, we observe maximum number of rasoushadhas added. Bhavana with kashaya of drugs listed in the formula to potentiate it .later we see 16 parts of that kasturi, 16 parts of pacchakarpooram added and prepared into vati form in the dose of one gunja 125 mg

In the preparation of Hemagarbhapotalirasa (kshaya prakaranam) we observe gandhaka is added 14 parts in a given yoga, and in other yoga equal quantity of Gandhaka. Such drugs probably selected by the author confident about the drug clinical efficacy add up in equal quantity in order to potentiate the action in achieving clinical success .This practice se is seen among the vaidyas of Andhra Pradesh even today.

While describing about kanta vallabharasa. We see proportionately the drug quantity reduced by 2 parts eg. Kantabhasma 16 parts, Teekshna bhasma 14 parts, manduram 12 parts, tankanam 10 parts and manishila added to it. We find 66 parts each of padarasa and gandhaka added to it in order to potentiate it.

In sambhavirasa we find adding of maricha chaurna 10 times of summation of drugs and 5 times of vatsanabhi.

Ekamurtiras yoga mentioned for sita jwara, in which suddha musaka pashanam is to be boiled in madhu for 1yama then this material is collected, dried and made into fine powder form administered in the dose of canaka . He claims after intake of this medicine. Vomiting takes place then only seetajwara gets subdued.

We observe that ksharas and lavanas have been used in abundance. In udayabhaskararasa we see many kshara and lavana and Trikatuka added in abundance In kshara tamra rasa mentioned in sula prakaranam we find kshara (cincaksara) in abundance (8parts) . Agni kumara rasa mentioned in sulaprakaranam we find adding of marica 8parts .

In the preparation of sankhavatukamulu (ajirna roga prakaranam). We see the predominance of chincha ksharam, aswata kshara, snuhi kshara, apamarga kshara arkakshara added in abundance along with pancha lavan also in abundance.

In chitrakadivatukamulu we observe that lavanam and pancha lavanam are separately mentioned. Under Vata prakaranam we observe khsaras and pancha lavanas are used in abundance.

In the preparation of vatarirasa, it is abundant in padarasa (8 pala) gandhaka (8 pala) and added with 14 palas of Jaggery.

In the making of sparsarirasa we observe the practice of keeping the medicine in a pot smeared with ghee.

In the preparation of Jateephaladi putapakam, dadimabeeja are added to ahiphena, gandhaka etc and these are again put in the fruit of pomegranate and coated with flour then cooked until it attains pakwa state.

In Vatarirasa we observe the ingredients parada, gandhaka, Triphala, citraka guggulu added by increasing one in succession i.e 1, 2, 3, 4, 5 parts respectively.

This churna given mardana in eranda thaila and abhyanjana also done with eranda thaila.

We see a even order in the making of sunthee churna i.e. sunthichurnam taken 21 tulas and fried in 21 tulas of ghee.

In Satavari thailam & Maha Vishagarbha thailam we see maximum number of ingredients probably not mentioned by any Ayurvedic text.

Mashadi tailam mentioned in vataprakaranam we find ajamamsa and tila tailam in abundance. These thailas are very much praised by the author that apart from treating vataroga, they strengthen the reproductive organs and improvess virility in male.

In the preparation of vatakulantaka thailam (vata prakaranam) resoushadhas i.e. parada, gandhaka, Talaka etc. are made into paste and applied to a cloth and twisted to form as wick than immersed in oil .It is removed and burnt at the end of it and when oil that dribbles collected in a crucible coated by ghrita. This is again applied to betel leaf and is given to the patient to eat to relieve the disease.

Under Vata prakaranam, the preparation of rasonapaka, the external layer of lasuna is removed and allowed to soak. On the next day it is cooked in milk of 246 tula, afterwards other ingredients like rasna vasa, guduci, devadaru are added. After having cooled it is added with honey.

Kuberapaka in which kuberaksha bija added prastha 768 gm along with other drugs, and considered very effective in all vatarogas and also considered vajikaraka and sthanya vardhaka.

In the making of lasunpaka we find lasuna (allium sativum bulb) added 1 prastha along with 4 pala of milk and other vatahara dravya and avaleha prepared. It is indicated in all vata disorders particular in painful conditions.

Deepyadi churnam and Kalyanaras (Sankha kshara), Triptisagararasa comprise number of kshara.

In the preparation of Kachoradichurnam we see pancha lavana and kshara are given importance. In (grahani prakaranam) . Chitrakadi Vatukamulu kshara and lavana are used abundantly.

In the preparation of Kankayana gutika we observe increasing pattern of the quantity of the ingredients pippalee pippalee mulam, modi charyam chitrakam sonthi, yava ksharam are added in the order taken 1, 2, 3, 4, 5, 6, 7, 8 palas respectively. Bhallataka 1 pala and surana taken twice of it. Likewise peculiar order is seen. (ref no146).

Madhupakwa hareetaki:

हरीतकीनां च शतं डोलायंत्रे शनैः पचेत् ॥ १५३ ॥ सुस्विन्नं गोमयैर्नीरे संसृष्टे तु पुनस्ततः । पश्चात्क्षुद्रशलाकाभिश्छिद्रितं तत्समं ततः ॥ १५४॥ शतं पलानां मधुनो वस्त्रपूतं विनिक्षिपेत् । स्निग्धभांडे विनिक्षिप्य क्षौद्रं देयं तथा तथा ॥ १५५ ॥ यथायथा हि मधुनो जलत्वं याति निश्चितम् । पुनर्देयं मधु तथा यावन्नायातिविक्रियाम् ॥ १५६॥

In the preparation of madhupakwa hareetaki a formulation of sangrahani prakaranam, 100 Hareetaki are cooked in gomayaras of dolayantra. Later these are removed and pricked and kept in a pot having ghee application. Fresh Honey is poured into this pot everyday, later pippali lavanga, Triphala etc are added. 1 haritaki is to be taken early in the morning.

Author is particular about what type of metal to be used for stirring and also the untensil to be used in the preparation of given medicine. Many a time he advises iron and copper metals.

In the making of suvarna rasa parpati, sutam svarna bhasma given mardana with nimba Drava added to gandhaka kept in lohapatra and stirred with badara stick and cooked. After that the substance is poured on banana leave which is placed evenly on cow dung and allowed to dry and later made into powder.

While describing rasakriya for eyes (ntra roga prakaranam) he advises the paste of the drugs to be kept in copper container and triturated with copper pestle by adding appropriate quantityof nimbaptra swarasa and varti is to be prepared. They are indicated in arma and sukla.

In netra roga prakaranam we come across another reference This is as follows Jambeeraswarasa kept in Iron utensil and to solidify it mardana is done with iron irod.

In the preparation of deepikadi thailam it is said that brihat panchamula measuring eight inches are tied up with silk cloth and the end is slowly burnt to get thailam.

The preparation of khandava churnam (Aruchiprakaranam) we find a set of drugs like talisapatra, cavya nagakesara etc., each taken as one part, another set of drugs like pippali cinca, citraka etc ., each taken 2 parts, likewise another set of drugs ela, amlavetasa, ajamoda etc., taken 3 parts and are added. Majority of the yogas are added with honey or juice of promegranate or sarkara (36 parts) in abundance to bring taste to the patient .

In khandava churnam and yavanee khanda churnam sarkara is added 45 pala and 64 pala respectively.

In the formulation of nasya we find that the administered medicine macerated either with water or milk or breast milk eg. Hareeta kyadi nasyam, Dadima pushpadi nasyam. 10 parts maricha churnam added in the preparation of Bhutankussaras.

In the preparation of lokanatha Pottaliras (Kasa prakaranam) . We see the practice of keeping kajjali in a box made up of tamra, and this box is kept in the middle of salt filled pot. This is put on fire after sealing it and cooked for 8 yama. This medicine is added with nabhi and maricha.

Likewise we see that he adds up sarkara, Jaggery, Chitramula, honey, ghee pippalee mula churnam maricha churnam to get the required affect. Even some times we see the adding up mutton soup of Tittiri bird added with ghee (dasamula ghritam) . While preparing the medicine Eranda mula churnam added in Kulatthadi Kashayam.

स्तन्येन मक्षिका विष्ठां नस्यं वालक्तकोंबुना । योज्यं हिक्काभिभूतेभ्यस्स्तन्यं वा चंदनान्वितम् ॥

In patalee yoga we observe swarnabhasma added to pataliphalarasa. In madhuka nasyam we observe the excreta of makshika added with breast milk and given as nasya to relieve hikka.

Pippalayadi loha added with lohabhasma taken in equal quantity to other drugs for example in sunthee ghritam we see rasabhasma, tamarabhasma and lohabhasma added in equal quantities. In most of his yogas herbs and minerals are added up depending on the clinical condition

In the making of garudanjana we observe the human skull, egg, broken pieces of pot are also included as ingredients

In the preparation of netranjanam we see nagabhasma, paradabhasma, lohabhasma, vatsanabhi are added as ingredients.

In Rasanjanadyanjana (netra roga prakaranam) Kurmaprista, manishila are amongst the ingredients.

It is interesting to note that pippali's are kept amidst of dried chaga sakrit to prepare anjana. Souveeranjana preparation too we come across unusual methods as follows. Sauveeram burnt seven times and dipped in Triphala Kashaya for 7 times to cool it, and again cooled it in breast milk for 7 times. We find some times the medicine kept in a shell and sealed and later given puta (Laghulokeswararasa).

In the preparation of lepa (Anda vidradhi prakaranam) mamsarasa, ghrita, taila are also been used. In another yoga we find Triphala are burnt and the soot added with honey to prepare leha (upadamsa prakaranam).

In the making of Agnimukha lavanam we see equal quantity of saindhava lavanam added.

In the formulation of vardhamana pippali (udara roga) author uses increasing pattern of adding of pippali.i.e. 3 pippali, 5 pippali, 7pippali, 10 pippali churna in the treatment vatarakta, kshaya.

In Vasanta Kusumakararasa a formulation mentioned for kshaya all the ingredients are uniformly mixed and 7 bhavanas are given in each liquid i.e vasa and candana.

In the preparation of krimimudgararasa we observe increasing pattern of drug add up ie rasa, gandhaka, ajamoda, vayuvidanga and vishamusti beeja added in 1, 2, 3, 4, 5, parts respectively

In the preparation of rasaushadha, lepa, ghrita taila etc author has taken liberty in adding up dravyas in abundanbce which he considers to be clinically proven and efficacious. Thus, some times he did not follow the strict norms of the preparation of formulations mentioned in other ayurvedic texts, and also, he has given new names to his newly formulated yogas.

Narikela jalam is given much importance in the yogas of mutrakrichra (ref narikela ghrita, mootrakrichra prakaranam) . This narikela ghrita is prepared by narikela jalam, kusmanda and satavari, jivaka, rshabhaka, yastimadhu etc.This is one among the new preparations of the author.

There is another practice of adding of churna in kashayam to potentiate the formulations and also to suit individual needs. Kashayams are sometimes added with bhasma, sarkara and honey. Dasamula kashayam and gokshuradi kashayams are added with shilajitu bhasma and sarkara to treat urinary disorders.

While describing icchabhedhirasam a formulation mentioned for udara roga, author states that this yoga will induce virechana number of times corresponding to the number of times of ushna jala taken .

In medoroga prakaranam lohabhasma is given importance. Hence we find number of formulations consisting lohabhasma as the main ingredient.

Paradadi churnam (chardhi prakaranam) given bhavana with chandana kashaya and administered after adding honey and maricha churnam. Adding up of madhu and maricha churnam appears to be a common phenomenon with the author .

Under swasa prakaranam we see the new add up yoga bharangee guda rasayanam.

In Maha parangyadi rasayanam a new yoga of the author, in this phiranga twak (it is used twice) and it is added up with gandhakam and rasa sindhuram (prameha prakaranam) .In this yoga we find that there is a traditional practice of worshipping visvaksena dhanvantari, later brahmanas, and also a share to vaidya is given. Varunadi kashayam a formulation mentioned for mutraghata added with yavaksharam then administered (An alkali preparation from the plant of barley).

Chitrakadi kashayam added with saindhava lavanam and administered. In dwandwaja shula, kashayams are added with sarkara and madhu.

Suryavartiras (Swasa prakarana) padarasa gandhaka added with maricha churnam.

In Kapitthadi Kashayam we observe that it been added with Erandamula churnam to enhance the effect.

Palasamula powder triturated with tandulodaka and used as upanaha. For the treatment of external lepa for galaganda.

Then 1 part of Chandra prabhava rasa is to be mixed with 10 parts of bakuchi and mardana to be done with gomutra in order to potentiate it.

Uddhamakhya rasa another contribution by the author. In this suddharasa macerated with sankhapushpi and sarpakshirasa, and equal to rasam jaipala (strong cathartic) is added .It is considered best for pitta gulma.

Gulmodara gajarati rasa another new formulation by the author .In this description he mentions "streenam jalodaram hanti".It cures ascites (jalodaram) of female is a new clinical condition (in cancer ovary ascites is an inevitable condition).

Another reference of new clinical condition is found in hridroga prakaranam (ref 155).

It states that krimi which are incurable dwell in hridaya will fall down with the consumption of vayuvidanga and kostu mixed with gomutrapana.

Dhupa -Describing about dhupa (Sitajwara, jwara prakaranam) we find certain odd things also in the making of dhupa. They include Khara vista (excreta of ass), kakapaksha (The wings of crow), lasuna twak, suskagouli (dried lizard), excreta of dog, and the hair of goat.

In **Ajadi dhupam** we find goat's hair as ingredient. In ulooka paksha dhupam the ingredients include owls wings. Other general ingredients include mahishaksa guggulu, vasa, kostu, nimba, arka, sarjarasa etc.

In the preparation of dhupa we find that the following such as saranga vista (excreta of deer), kola vista (the excreta wild boar) the sikhi pincha (feathers of peacock), the serpents (cast skin) dried chamaeleon, all put together and the powder is administered as dhupa.

There is practice of macerating churna with hot water and administered as nasya (Marichyadinasyam, sannipata prakaranam).

In the preparation of anjanam also we see certain specialties like the soot resulted due to burning of spider net is mentioned in Jwara prakaranam.

In some clinical conditions honey or oil alone is administered as nasya.

Describing Arkamuladi dhumam it is advised to take tambulam or milk after swallowing dhuma.

Administering and dose of the formulations:

Depending on the clinical condition, author some times adjusted the dose, for eg. Karsha in the morning and half karsha in the evening. Probably to suit the digestive capabilities of a particular time.

We observe another mode of administration such as Administering of the medicine in the morning for 21 days. Advised to take early in the morning for 21 days.

Under shula prakaranam we get the reference for vata shula it is recommended to apply shigru lepa over the umbilical area. Rjika brassica juncea and sigru moringa triturated in gotakra and applied on umbilicus.

They were cautious while administering cathartics to patients.

It is evident by observing a note on Kustadi thaila of gulmaroga prakaranm that the medicine is to be taken once in four days but not everyday.

There is another practice of taking medicine i.e. first morsel to be mixed with medicine and administered.

Eg: Samudradi churnam (udararoga prakaranam).

In Vranaroga prakaranam when we go through hasti dantadi lepam, it is said that hastidanta macerated on stone with water and if applied just as a drop it causes bhedana of vrana is surprising.

To adminster churna as nasya they macerated in arka ksheera added with kajjali then nasya is given. In sannipata prakaranam it is to note that Easwari root and the seeds of eswari are added with equal quantity of maricha churna and given as nasya.

Ahiphenam: In vaidya chintamani we find number of references of Ahiphenam. We observe much yoga are added with ahiphenam. It is particularly used in the diseases of atisara (diarrhoea) and in the conditions of sula (pain). It is evident by the following references.

In suddhi prakaranam it is said ahiphena tied up gajakarnadala (balurakkasi aku) and to cook in dola yantra for its suddhi. The following are the yogas having Ahiphenam as its parts.

In Daradadiputapakam, ahiphenam is added four parts for 1 part of darada.

In the making of Kanakasundararasa the drugs are given maceration in Vijayee Drava. In the making of grahani gaja kesarirasam, ahiphenam is added equal to other parts in summation.

In the preparation of agsti sutaraja, ahiphenam is added to a larger extent. In the makingof Vajrakavata rasa, ahiphenam is added and all the drugs are given mardana with.

In the making of vata vidhwamsini rasam and sameera gaja kesari rasa ahiphenam is added. All these formulation are popular till today, and are very much prescribed by ayurvedic physicians in particular Andhra Pradesh owing to its time tested assuring results.

Loha/Manduram.

In vaidyachintamani we find loha is given much importance. In much yoga loha bhasma is the main ingredient, and also described this metal vividly. The following are the contributions with respect to loha and manduram. In pandu prakarana we come across many references indicates that they possess good knowledge about loha to combat bloodlessness of pandu. The following are references.

1) "Kaasmeera loha sakalena vasrutam tanmalena ... pandu gada sopha kamila"

2) Rasam gandham varaschata ... visham vangabhrakanta teekshna mandam ..... Samansam sakalena Trigunam purana kittam

The use of kanta bhasmam, ukkubhasma, ayobhasma is seen in this yoga and also we see manduram is added three times to the summation of other ingredients

The following rasoushadhas prepared by him posses lohabhasma. They are lohasundararas, pandunigraha rasa. In panchkola mandooram 12 palas of manduram is added. In mahamanduram an exclusive preparation by him. We find 10 palas of loha kittam is being used. In Rasa sindhura bhushana lohabhasma is added 10 times to the ingredients. Equal quantities of rasa, gandhakam and lohabhasm are added in pandvarirasa. In loha sundararas we observe Rasa, loha bhasam and gandhaka are taken 1, 2, 3 parts respectively. In one yoga we see 12-pala mandura being used. Among the best mandura is Narayana mandura in which equal quantity of manduram is added to other medicine in summation. Describing madhumandooram we can note that mandooram is taken prastham and also it is written that it produces blood "gruheetwa bhishakprastha mandura ...... Janakorudhirasyasha" (Pandu prakaranam).

There is one mandura preparation (vibheetaka – lavanam) administered adding vibheetaki and saindhava lavanam, an excellent contribution by him. This praised by the author so much that no other medicine can cure pandu than this yoga. Krutvagni varnam – pandvamayaghnam nahikinchidanyat".

In another mandura preparation which is added with kirata etc drugs. Lohabhasma added equal quantity to all of the other drugs in summation. Another yoga in which mandooram is cooked in gomutra, and its churna taken along with Jaggery.

Another variety of mandooram mentioned by the author is Hamsamandooram. In this yoga Mandooram is cooked in gomootra taken eight times of it.

Siddhamandooram another contribution by the author. In this manduram of 8 pala is cooked in gomutram taken 64 times after that its choorna is added with other panduhara drugs.

In mandura vataka we see the mandooram is taken twice the quantity of other drugs mixed. Darvadi Vatukamulu, punarnavadi vatukamulu, mandura vajra vatukamulu in all these yogas manduram shares major part. (Manduram is added 4 palas, 2 palas and 6 palas respectively) . Other yogas of mandura importance are navayasa churnam, Triphaladi lahyam (8 parts of loha churna taken), chinchadi lehyam (Chinchapatra 100 pala, ayasam (loham 50 pala), loham 3 palam, manduram 2 palas are added. In yoga laghuchinchadi lehyam we see the similar ingredients like chincha patra (100 it is added with lohabhasma 4 palas. Describing lohamritarasam 18 pala of lohabhasma is added.

Author has formulated yogas with loha bhasma, manduram to suit different kinds of clinical conditions basing on dosha and prakriti. This many varities of manduram are not described at one place in any of the text, and it is not just adding of manduram in yoga but added almost equal to the quantity to other drugs.

Kitta: Iron when burnt in the furnace the excreta that emerges is known as kitta. We get the characteristics and classification such as mundaha kitta, teekshnaja kitta and kantaja kitta. Kitta is considered best if it is 100 years old and medium if it is 80 years old and less than 60 it is considered as inferior. It is mentioned that the kitta has to be kept in furnace and blown to become red to be known as manduram.

In Ajeerna Prakaranam while mentioning about Sanjeevani gutika states that if one pill is given with ardraka rasa relieves ajeerna. If 2 pills are administered cures Visuci, 3 pills are given cure posion, and if 4 pills are given relieves sannipata. Clinical indications cured depending on the number of pills administered is amazing.

2) While explaining about Kshudasagara Vatukamulu (Ajeerna Prakaran) he indicates that these 2 pills should be consumed along with either 5 lavanga or 7 lavanga in order to get cured from Ajeerna. This kind of specification 5 lavanga or 7 lavanga is interesting.

3) To eat apupa prepared from kalka akhuparni dala along with sauveeraka destroys krimi is a novel way of administering medicine.

4) Mere drinking of Haridra mixing with either of the mutra such as gomutra, naramutra or with puranaghrita destroys all poisons.

5) While describing ardhanareeswara ras, author states that if this yoga is given as drops in the ear relieves one from parshwa Jwara

कतकस्य फलं शंखं सैंधवं त्रयूषणं सिता ।। ११० ।।

फेनो रसांजनं क्षौद्रं विडंगानि मनःशिला । कुक्कुटांडकपालं च खल्वमध्ये विनिक्षिपेत् ।। १११ ।। सर्वमेतत्समं कृत्वा नारीक्षीरेण पेषयेत् । तिमिरं पटलं काचमर्मशुक्रं व्यपोहति ।। ११२ ।।

कंडूक्लेदार्बुदं हन्ति मलं बाह्यं जयेत्ततः । (katakadyanjana)

कणा छागशकृन्मध्ये पक्वा तद्रसपेषिता । अचिरद्धन्ति नक्तांध्यं तद्वत्सक्षौद्रमूषणम् ।। १५७ ।। (kanadyanjana)

When we observe the preparation of anjanam, it is very strange to note that it contains the bones of human skull, phenam, iron bhasma, egg shell

and manishila macerated in Jeera Kashaya and applied in the eyes will relieve kusumam (white patch on cornea) even if it is present since birth is amazing.

Likewise, describing girikarikadyanjana, shiladayanjana, Maha narikeladyanjanam, author claims that with the administration of these anjana the person gets back his sight and will be able to see the stars even in the day time "Divanakshatra darsanam". But taking note of the ingredients such as godanta, kukkutanda kapala makes one deter from using them as application of the eye.

Author mentioning the preparation of kanadyanjana mentions that Pippali is to be placed in the Ajamala and heated, there after this Pippali is mixed again with Ajamala swarasa then triturated and administered in the form of Anjana.

7) Chinnacharlagadda, bhringaraja, Trikatuka, taken them in a cloth and squeezed them in the ear insects will be expelled It is amazing to note that while describing

Badabanalarasa he says that 7 days of its administration cures eighteen types of kusta, 6 months of its administration makes one attain sareera siddhi and 1 year of administration makes one similar to god easwara .And also it is said in his mutra and pureesha tamra, swarna gets produced. . In these preparations gandhaka and vakuchi are given importance.

In masurika prakaranam there is indication that flies cause disease and they should be flown away by nimba patra and sakha. We also get reference that masurika patient should be kept in isolation and to observe quarantine period.

In gala ganda prakaranam we come across unique and strange preparations, which are considered to cure, galagandam is worth noting. They are as follows:

1) Loha Kitta kept in a pot containing mahishee mutra for one long month later macerated and given gaja puta and the powder taken with honey to cure galaganda.

2) Water preserved in ripen bitter alabu for 7 days, then such water is given to drink cures galaganda.

3) Appropriate quantity of Bida and Saindhava lavana added to Jeerna Karkaruka phala swarasa and administered as nasya will cure galaganda without any doubt.

4) It is said that Vishnu kranta jata kalka added up with sarkara and madhu cures parinama shula if taken for 7 days.

5) Gorocana bile ox, haridra, manjista, ghrita, gairika are triturated with goats milk and applied over the face in the early morning increases the glow of the face .

6) . Under vrana roga prakaranam ayorajadi lepa it is mentioned that loham, kaseesam, triphala, lavanga and

daruharidra rubbed together and applied imparts new skin at the place of vrana.

7) Gandhadi lepa: Powder of equal quantities of gandhaka, manishila, shunti, vayuvidanga given mardana with krikala raktam (blood of sarat) girigit and applied arbuda gets destroyed immediately.

8) Palasamula lepa : Palasamula powder is macerated with tandulodaka and applied on the ears subdues gala ganda.

9) In trishna prakaranam while mentioning about rasadi gutika it is mentioned that parada bhasma and rajita bhasma are mixed together and chewed relieves trishna.

10) Mentioning about visuchi kashayam in ajeerna prakaranam it is said that urine of the child when boiled and added with pippali churnam not only cures visuchi but also increases digestive power.

ANUPANAS MENTIONED IN VAIDYACINTAMANI

Anupana is that material which is consumed along with food or medicine. It can increase the palatability of the food or medicine, can improve the digestion and absorption and also act as a vehicle, which carries the drug to their target site.

Apart from the usual anupana the following are different varieties of anupana mentioned by him in Vaidyachinatamani as follows. In the brackets name of theformulation given.

Jaggery water, Usnodaka (hot water); Seetodakam; Ghee added with trikatu; Rice gruel added with honey; Sour butter milk; Honey or ghee; Honey or ghee Kshaya; Katutrayanupanam; Curd; . Uda and kshaudra; seetodaka; Goats urine; Honey added to rice gruel; Mahisha takra; Jagerry, butter milk; Godugdha; Tambulam; Gomutram; Goghritam; Butter milk; Sarpakshirasa kashayam; Arkamulakshaya or lasuna swarasa; Erandathailam, gomutra, goghrita; Ushnambu, goghrita; Draksha hareetaki kwatham; Draksha pathya kwatham. Ardrakarasa, khandasarkara; madya; Dadhi madya or mamsarasa;

Duration of treatment: Those days the patients were asked to follow the prescription for a specified period. And also, they were so confident in telling about the prognosis of the disease, and also in certain clinical conditions they could foresee and said that the medicine to be used for specified period and the patient will be cured of the disease, or he or she will die of the disease. It is also said if the patient gets recovered from the disease, then it is said that he will live for 100 years is amazing. The following are examples to show the variation of the period of treatment for each of the formulation they are as follows.

Grahanee kavata rasa administered for 1 month; Kshara tamra rasa for 40 days; Shadaseeti guggulu for 1 year (vata prakaranam).

They could identify some of the disease as self limiting disease such as masurika etc. they have restricted the span of treatment limited to few days. Even for lepa also they have stipulated time schedule. In kusturoga prakaranam one churna prescribed for sweta kustu indicated to take the medicine for six months.

While describing pasupati krita churnam (kustu roga prakaranam) it is mentioned to take for seven months. Describing about Jathyadivatukamulu (Meha prakaranam) we see the indication to take the medicine for 40 days.

Describing maha chinchadi lehyam (pittaprakaranam) author indicates to take the medicine for one month.

Author advises Trilokyadambararasa (udararoga) to take the medicine for 21 days.

Seetarirasa (Seetapitta prakarana) is advised to take the medicine for 30 days.

While prescribing drastic purgatives the patients were asked to take once in 4 days. Generally the patients were asked to take medicines twice a day irrespective of the duration of the treatment.

General dose patterns mentioned vaidyachintamani:

We get the following dose patterns prescribed for the patients in vadiyachintamani. They are, Valla, gunja, masha, mudga, chanaka, nishka, tila, udumbara sama, varaha, panitala, karsha, Badara (seetapitta prakaranam), Bolus (Daradadi putapaka), Maricha, Aksha Tula and marjalapada.

References of panchakarma in vaidyachintamani

Notes: *Panchakarma is a method of cleansing the body of all the unwanted waste after lubricating it. Panchakarma are 5 (five) in number. Panchakarma treatment is unique in the sense that it includes preventive, curative and promotive actions for various diseases.*

Five Karmas

The body can be divided on the basis of the parts that need cleansing. Head, GIT (gastro- intestinal system), upper and lower. The five main Karmas to cleanse the complete body are

1) Vamanam (therapeutic emesis) - induced vomiting helps clear the upper gastro till the duodenum (end of stomach) and part of the respiratory tract.

2) Virechanam (purgation) - Induced purgation clears the lower gastro from the duodenum (end of stomach) till the exit.

3) Anuvasana (enema using medicated oil) - Oil enema helps lubricate the rectal area and take out all the lipid soluble waste out through the anus.

4) Nasyam - nasal instillation of medicated substances helps clear the respiratory tract and para-nasal sinuses.

5) Asthapana Vasti (Therapeutic Decoction Enema) - decoction enema cleanses the area from the transverse colon till the anus.

The complete process of Panchakarma consists of three steps.

A) Poorva Karma, which is the preparatory procedure required before the main procedure to enable a person to receive the full benefits of the main treatment. It consists of two main processes – Snehan (oleation) and Swedan (fomentation) . These methods help to dislodge the accumulated poisonous substances in the body, thus preparing them for their complete removal.

B) Pradhan Karma or the main procedure: On completion of the first step, it is decided which of these are to be done depending upon the proximity of the waste. An increased level of upper respiratory tract waste shall call for Vamana. Similarly, a lower gastro accumulation of waste calls for a Virechanam.

C) Paschaat Karma or the post-therapy dietary regimen to restore the body's digestive and absorptive capacity to its normal state.

Raktamokshana is an effective blood purification therapy that decreases an increased level of Pitha Dosha. As a result, all this treatment relieves all Pitta-related diseases. This blog aims to cover the types and benefits of this ancient Ayurvedic treatment.

Sushruta had cited Raktamokshana as one of the five purification methods in Panchakarma. One can divide this procedure into two parts, and these are:

1. Shastra Visravana

This type of Raktamokshana procedure uses metallic instruments. Furthermore, Ayurvedic practitioners have divided Shastra Visravana into two subcategories, and they are:

Siravyadhana- we know this method as venipuncture in the modern day. One uses a syringe to remove impure blood from a person's veins in this method.

Pracchana- In this method, a physician uses a blade or scalpel to make superficial incisions on this skin. This way, blood exudes out through several superficial incisions.

Furthermore, a sub-type of this method is Alabu Pracchana, where an Ayurvedic practitioner uses a bottle gourd or any other conical-shaped vegetable. These vegetables are used to create a vacuum over an incision. Many believe this technique to be the forerunner of Chinese and European wet cupping techniques, which appeared many years later.

2. Anushastra Visravana

This type of Raktamokshana Panchakarma does not involve any metallic instruments. Anushastra Visravana is also divided into two sub-categories, which are:

Jalaukavacharana- In this method, an Ayurvedic practitioner applies leeches to specific areas of a person's body.

Shrungavacharana- this method uses a cow's horns. The Vata conditions are also treated alongside Pitta imbalances in this procedure.

In vaidyachintamani panchakarma was not given proper place in the treatment of any given disease .In addition to that even tridosha vivechana for given disease is also not given importance.No drug or formulation was mentioned in terms that cause aggravation or palliation of dosha .Vasti almost mentioned nowhere except in the chapter on amlapitta, but rare references of panchakarma reveal that in those days they were well aware of panchakarma therapies .We get mere indication of names of the procedures of panchakarma but not going in details of panchakarma methods, its drugs, dosage shedule procedures of panchakarma .It is strange to find the mention of panchakarma while mentioning of pathya and apathya of each disease.

The following are the references pertaining to panchakarma in vaidya chintamani.

There is indication of vamana, virechana and raktamokshana . One after the other in the above said preceding order the patient is instructed to undergo if the disease do not come under control with the internal medication. There is no mention of time duration, dose complications etc with reference to Panchakarma .

He indicates drakshadi kashayam in the conditions of sleshma pittam, but for pitta sleshmam he advises virechanam and vamanam.

While discussing about the treatment of amlapitta he advises vamana in the beginning and later virechana then anuvasana vasti . And if the disease of longer duration niruha vasti is recommended.

If dosha are pervading in the upper part of the body then vamana is indicated, virechana indicated for doshas pervading the lower part of the body.

In the disease seeta pitta prakaranam abhyangam, a purva karma of panchakarma is indicated with katu thailam.Swedam with ushnodakam, later vamanam with patolarista or vasa kashayam is indicated. Then virechana is advised with triphala, guggulu and pippali later mahatiktaka ghritam is given as drink. Lastly raktamokshana is employed.

In vata rakta prakaranam rakta mokshanam is mainly indicated. Depending on dosa vitiation jalouka, alabu and shringa are administered.He specially mentions sneha yukta virechanam in pittadhika vatarakta. And in bahya vata rakta he advocates abhyanga, parisheka and also upanaha.

In udararoga prakaranam Narayanachurnam is indicated for virechana to those patients who have attained laghu kosta with pachana, swedana therapies.

In kaphaja galaganda sweda kriya upanaha kriya are indicated.

In all types of galaganda vamanam and siro virechanam are indicated.

In the disease visarpa, virechana is indicated with trivrith and triphala.

Vamana is to be induced with chakota rasa.

While discussing about agantuka vrana raktamokshana is indicated

Vamanam is advocated in amasayastha rudhiram and virechana in pakwashayastha rudhiram. To remove sukadosa vamanam and rakta mokshanam are indicated .

In ajagallika rakta mokshanam is indicated. (Ref kshudra roga prakaranam) . We find the mention of sneha and sweda in the disease avapatika .

In surya varta, sira vyadha (diseases of head) nasya, virechanam, are indicated.In anantavata sira vedhana indicated .In pittaja siroroga virechanam is indicated. In kaphaja siroroga sweda etc., karma are indicated. In sannipataja siroroga sirovasti, sirodhumam, sirovirechanam, swedam are indicated.

It can be concluded that in those days the physicians were well aware of the procedures of panchakarma, but they did not follow them in its rigid sense, but have administered them whenever necessitated. Vaidyacintamani did not mention the detailed procedures of panchakarma, the drugs to be used in the pancha karma treatment, their dosage, purvakarma of pancha karmas, preparation of the patient before panchakarma procedures, in what diseases panchakarma procedures should be adopted. What are the eligibility criteria; complications, knowledge about the tools etc were not described. Probably this book served as a ready reckoner of internal medicine with formulations for medical practitioners who were already well versed in the procedures of panchakarma.It can be predicted that in those days panchakarma procedures were routinely followed by the general public and also done by the physicians .It should be noted that the description of pathya, apathya given at the end of each chapter on disease .Almost in all of them it is mentioned that which panchakarma procedures should be under taken, and also about procedures of panchakarma which are contraindicated.

The following are some examples in support of it.

Describing pathya of vata rakta, the following panchakarma procedures such as in uttana vatarakta abhyanjana, seka,, upanaha, lepa indicated. And in gambheera vatarakta snehapana, vastikarma, rechana, raktamokshana, abhyanga with satadhouta ghritam and avasechanam with aja dugdham etc are advised.

PATHYA AND APATHYA OF DISEASES

In common the following food and activities considered as pathya.

Tanduliyaka, vastuka, balmulaka, parpata (parviflora lam), patola (trichosanthes dioica), tilasaka, guducipatra (tinospora cordiofolia), kalsha, nimba pushpa, (citrus lemon) marica (variety vegetable), darvikadalam, jivanti, changeri, sunisannaka etc vegetables are considered as Pathya

Mudga (phaseolus rodiatus) masura, (lens culinaris chanaka, kulatha mudga yusa are satmya.

Lavapakshi, kapinjala, hirana, prusata, kalkuccha, and mrga are considered satmya, where as meat of sarasa, kruch, shikir, tittir and kukkuta is satmya brintak, pilu, karkota, patola, kattilaka (bitter gourd) etc., fruit vegetables ae to be given in the treatment of jwara, one year old rice or dhanya.roti prepared from 2 year old godhuma (wheat) .

While describing jirna jwara pathya are virechana, anjanam and nasya, dhumapan, anuvasana vasti swedana etc. Describing agantuka jwara langhana is contra indicated. And also swasthivacana, pitta shamaka karma, japa, homa etc daiva vyapashraya chikitsa mentioned .

Apathya in taruna jwara: bath, virecana vyayama, vyavaya, kashaya, day time sleep mamsa takra, sura, krodha are to be prohibited. Viruddhannapana brushing, germinated seeds, abhashyanda padartha are prohibited.

The following are some of the important pathya and apathy of important diseases.

Kshaya: Mrdu sodhan to reduce dosa vikriti, a godhuma, mudga, canaka, sasti dhanya, agoat meat, butter, cows ghee, milk meat of mamsahari jantu, moon rays, pakwa mamsa churna, madhura padartha, sitala vayu sevana, wearing of onaments containing mukta, homa, brahmana puja are pathya for kshaya patients.

Apathya: (kshaya) virecana, vegadharana, srama, swedana, anjana, jagarana, sahasakarma, ruksha annnapana visamasana, tambula, karbuja kulinga (meat of bird) lasuna, hingu, amal, tila, kashaya, katu patrasaka, viruddhahara, bimbi, vidahi dravya, Punarnava (boehavia difusa), are apathya in kshaya.

Pathya in pandu, kamala and kumbha kamala halimaka:

Vamana, virecana, purabna yavagodhuma, sali, mudga, tuvar (redgram) masura yusa (soup made up of lens culinaris), jangala jantu mamsa rasa patola, kushmanda taruna, kadalipahala jivanti lepatadeniareticulate guduchi matyakshi, dronapushpi, vartaka ripened mango bimbi, shringi, gomutra, ghrta, navanita, candana, nagakesara, lohabhasma kasaya dravya kesar all these are considered pathya according to dosa

Apathya:

Raktamokshana, dhumapana, vamana, vega dharana, swedana, coitus, simbiphala patra saka hingu, chitraka tambula amladravya dusta ahar, viruddha vihhar guru and vidahi ahar are considered apathya.

Sopha :

In the disease Sopha old rice, wheat, patola, tanduliyaka, punarnava, jharsi draksha, candana dadima, takra, madhu are pathya.

Apathya: Dadhi, nispava, katu padartha amla, vidahi padartha, madya tila are considered as apathya.

Atisara:

Pathya: vamana, langhana, nidra, purana sastirice, vlepi, laja, manda, dadhi, takra, navina kadaliphala, bilwa, ardraka, kapitha, bilwa, dadima, talaphala (palm tree fruit) vataphala, jayaphala, ahiphena, kutaja, kashaya rasa laghu and dipana anupana

Apathya: Snana, avagahana, abhyanga, guru snigdh ahara sevana, vyayama, navina dhanya, usna bhojana, coitus, fatigue, cinta, swedana, raktamokshana, jagarana, nasya, abhyanga, ruksha asatmya bhojana, nishpavaka, madhu ikshu, madya, draksha, amlavetasa, lasuna, newly collected water kasturi, lavana and amla dravya.

Vata vyadhi: Pathya: abhyanga, mardana, vasti, snehana, swedana, avagahana, angamardanavatasamaka kriya, samvahana, agnikarma, bhusayana, sirovasti, asana, taila, santarpana, brimhana, dadhimanda, nasya, ghrta, taila, vasa, majja, guggulu, grammya and anupa jantu mamsa sigru vartaka dadima, nagara, goksira, snigdoshna bhojana, dipana raktamokshan in case of twacavata, raktavata, siragatavata, raktamokshana is advised.

All these procedure are done according to the condition and bala.

Apathya: Cinta, jagarana, vegadharana, vamana, rama fasting, nivara dhanya, trna dhanya, rajamasa mudga, karira, jambu, singhada, pugiphala matsya, sitala jala gardabh shira, ksara, suska mamsa, horse roiding elephant riding, continuous walking taking food immediately after eating food, brushing, are apathya in vata roga.

Pitta prakaranam:

Pathya: Purana shalidhanya, patola, tanduliyaka, amalaki, vayastha, draksha, dadima candana are all pathya in 24 types of pitta.

Apathya: Dadhi, kshira guda, ghrta, masa, nispava, sarsapa, vidahi dravya, guru dravya.vyayama, krodha, atapa are apathya.

Kasa: Pathya: salishasthika dhanya, godhuma, mugdha, kulutha, ajadugdha, ajaghrta, bimbi, vartakamuli, jivanti, vastuka, nimbu, draksha, lasuan, laja sunthi, pippali.marica, usnajala, madhu.

Apathya: coitus, snigdha, madhura ahara, diwasvapna, dadhi, payasa, dhuma (inhalation of dust) are apathya.

Swasa:

Virecana, swedana, dhumrapana, vamana, diwasapna, kulutha, godhuma, rabit meat, peacock meat, tittira, lavaka bird meat, jangala jantu pakshi mamsa, dugdha, ghtrta, tanduliyaa, vastuka, ela, usnodaka, kapha vatahara bhojana and aushadhi.trikatu are considered pathya,

Apathya: Raktamokshana, air coming frm the east, newly collected rice, ajaghrta, kandamula (tubers), ruksha sita guru ahara, udgaravarodha, trsnavarodha, nasya, basti, srama (exercise) are considered apathya.

Aruci: vasti, virecana, vamana, dhumapana, kavala graha, danta dhavana, godhuma, mudga, adhaka, meat of rabit deer, pig fish, egg, kushmanda, dadima, floating water, kanji, madhutakra, ardraka, tinduka, kapitha, badruka, haritaki, marica, hingu, madhur amla tikta rasa dravya are pathya. Apathya: Vegavarodha, food which is not acceptable.

NAMES OF RISHIS WHO HAVE FORMULATED AND PROPAGATED A GIVEN YOGA.

One of the important contribution of vaidya chintamani is mentioning of names of those rishis who have prepared the yoga. This type of information though available scarcely in other texts but not to the extent mentioned in vaidya chintamani.The following is the list of names of rishis mentioned againist each yoga. References about names of rishis who prepared the yogas given in brackets.;

1) Sailushadi rasayanam (Aswini devatalu)

2) Mahasatavari thailam   (Sambamurthi).

3) Bhringamalaka thailam (Nithyanatha)

4) Mahabilvadi lehyam (Dhanwantari).

5) Avipattikara churnam (Agastyamuni)

8) Mahakalagnirudra ras   (Mahadevuni)

9) Maha kanaka sundara ras (Kasyapa mahamuni) etc

FREQUENTLY USED DRUGS IN VAIDYACHINTAMANI

A

Ajamoda (Apium leptophyllum); amalaki emblica officinalis)

ativisa aconitumheterophyllum), citraka (plumbagozeylanica)

jiraka (cuminumcyminum); patha (cissampelos pareira)

dhanyaka coriandrum sativum; jathamansi (Nardostachhys jatamansi)

yavani (trachyspermum ammi); pippalimula (piper longum)

nimbu (citrus limon); haritakki (terminalia chebula)

saindhava lavana (rock salt); vaca (acoros calamus)

sunthi (zingiber officinalis); marica (paper nigrum)

dalcini (cinnamom zeylnicum); bhringaraja (eclipta alba)

vatsanabha (aconitum chasmanthum); hingu (ferula foetida)

tila (sesamum indicum); haritaki (terminalia chebula)

sambhuka (spiral shell); guda (jaggery); satavari (asparagus recemosus);

dadhi (curd); dugdha (cows milk); goghrta (cows ghee);

haridra (curcuma longa); rudraksha (elaeocarpus sphaericus);

musta (cyperus rotundus); tumburu (zanthoxylum armatum);

Ela (elettaria cardamomum); cavya (piper retrofractum);

Bhallataka (semecarpus anacardium); kusta (saussurea lappa)

Swarnamakshika (chalcopyrite); pushkaramula (inula recemosa); vidannga (embelia ribes); gaja pippali (scindapsus officinalis);

Khadira (acacia catechu); madhu (honey);

Kuberaksha (caesalpinia bonduc trivrit operculina turpethum

Piluphala (salvodara persica); vaca (acorus calamus);

Arkamula (calotropis procera); snuhiksira (euphorbia meriifolia);

Punarnava (boerhavia diffusa); tumburu (xanthoxylum alatum)

Haritaki (terminalia chebula); yavakshara (hordeum vulggare);

Parada (mercury); aragvada majja (cassia fistula);

Sankhapushpi (convolvulus pluricaulis); jaiphala bija (processes croton tiglium jaipala bija croton tiglium vrkshamla (garcinia indica);

Patha (cissamelos pariera); amlavetasa (garcinia pedunculata);

hapusa (juniperus communis); Krishna jira (carum carvi);

Bharangi (clerodendrum serratum); Karanja (pongamia pinnata);

Devadaru (cidrus diodara); Tila ulam (sesamum indicum);

sauvarcala lavana (black salt); Vida lavana (vit salt);

Romaka lavana (sambar salt); Sauvarcala lavan (black salt)

Bijapura (citrus medica); Karanjapatra (pongamia pinnata); Gajacirbhata (citrullus colocynthis); Danti (baliospermum montanum);

Alabu bija (bottle guard lagenaria vulgaries); tuttha (blue vitriol)

Sati (hedychium spicatum); hingu (ferula foetida);

Jiraka (cuminum cyminum); Madhiphala (citrus medica);

Jambira (citrus limon); Cinca kshara (tamarindus indica);

Snuhi kshara (Euphorbia nerrifolia); Arkakshara (calotropis procera);

Nirgundi (vitex nigundo); Mundi (spharanthus indicus);

Sodhita sphatika (processed alum); Navasagara (ammonium chloride)

Sura kshara (potassium nitrate); Yastimadhu (glycyrrhiza glabra);

Vidarikanda (pueraria tuberosa); Phalsa (grewiaasiatica);

Trayamana (gentian kurroo); Dhamasa (fagonia Arabica);

Bhumyamalaki (phyllanthus amarus); Kumara (aloe barbansis);

Guduci (tinospora cordifolia); Candana (santalumalbum);

Kamala (nelumbo nucifera); Erandamula (ricinus communis);

Kampillaka (mallotus philippinensis); Matulunga (citrus medica);

Palasa (butea monosperma); Kustha (sassurea lappa);

Dadima (punica granthum); Dhamasa (fgonia Arabica);

Arjuna (terminalia arjuna); Nagabal (grewia hirsute);

Rasna (pluchea lanceolata); Yava (hordeum vulgare);

Kapitha (feronia limonia); kiratatikta (swertia chirata);

Daruharidra (berberis aristata); Haritaki (terminalia chebula);

Ajamoda (apium leptopilum); Patola (trichosanthes dioica);

Satapushpa (aneathum sowa); Ajagandha (cleome gynandra);

Kankusta (resin of mysore gambose tree); Visala (trichosanthes bracteata)

Satala (euphorbia pilosa); Swarnaksiri (argemone Mexicana);

Katuki (picrorhiza kurrora); Nilimula (indigofera tinetoria);

Kapardika (cowriest); Tankana (borax); Nepala bija (croton tiglium);

Talisapatra (abies webbiana)

Kampilaka (mallotus philippensis)

Girikarnika (clitorea ternatea); nilini (indigofera tinctoria)

Sankhapushpi (convolvuluspluricaulis)

Kantakari (solanum surattense)

Snuhi (euphorbia neriifolia)

Kaphardika (cowries); rohitaka (tecomella undulate)

Badarimula (zizypus jujube); Tumbaru (xanthoxylum armatum)

Indrayana (citrullus colocynthis); Brihati (solanum indicum)

Renuka (vitex agnus castus); Bala (sida cordifolia)

Vasa (adhtoda vasica); Gokshra (tribulus terrestris)

Aralu mula (ailanthus exsxcelsa); Putikaranja (caesalpinia crista)

Sigru (moringaoleifera); Pashana bheda (bergenia ciliate)

Padmaka (prunus cerasoides); Usira (vetiveria zizaniodes)

Nilkamala (nymphoea stellate); Laksa (laccifer lacca)

Gairika (red ochre); Kundaram (variety of grass)

Suska gomaya (dry cow dung); Indravaruni (citrullus colocynthis)

Langalimula (gloriosa superba); Iswarimula (aristolochia indica);

Musaka carma (skin of rat); Langali (gloriosa superba);

Tejapatra (cinamomun tamala); Karkatasrngi (pistacia chinensis);

Tagara (valeriana wallichii); Mundi (sphaeranthus indicus);

Kayaphala (myrica esculenta); Katuki (picrorhiza kurora);

Salaparni (desmodium gangeticum); bakuci psaralia caylifolia

Murva (marsedenia tenacissima); bakuci (psaralia carylifolia)

Saptaparna (alstoniascholaris); Indrayava (holarhena antidysenterica);

Manjista (rubia cordifolia); Nimba (Azadirachta indica);

Daruharidra (berberis aristata); cakramarda (cassia tora); Hrivera (coleus vettiveroides); Madhuka (madhuk aindica); Kokilaksha (asteracantha longifolia); Patola (trichosanthes dioica); Usira (vetiveriazizaniodes);

Raktachandana (ptterocarpus santalinus); Jambira (citrus lemon);

Visamusti (strychns nuxvomicš); Arka (calotropis procera); Dattura (datura metel); Karavira (nerium indicum); Karkataka sringi (pistacia integerrima);

Punarnava (boerhavia diffusa); Cakramarda (cassia tora); dalcini (cinnamomum zeylanicum); Nagakesara (mesua ferrea); Parpata (fumana ferviflora); Kacur (curcumazedoaria); Jyotismati (celastrus); Vyagranakha (capparis zeylanica); Padmaka (prunus cerasoides); tarkari (clerodendrum phlomidis); pilu (salvadora persica); nimbaphala azadirachta indica;

Asana (pterocarpus marsupium); gunja bija (abrus precatorius); kakamaci (solanum nigrum); dhamasa (fagonia Arabica); guggulu (commiphora wightii); kustha (sausurea lappa); prasarini (paderia foetida);

agnimantha (clerodendrum phlomidis); madhuka pushpa (madhuca indica);

Kucala (strychnos nuxvomica); bhallataka (semecarpus anacardium);

Himsra (capparis spinosa); vamsalocana (bambusa arundinaca);

Parpataka (fumaria purviflora); sarastri (alum); varuna (crateva nurvala);

Cirayata (swertia chirata); bilwa (aegle marmelos); kacura (curcuma zedoaria); varahi kanda (dioscoria); kushmanda (benincasa hispida); kadali musa (paraclisiaca); narangi (citrus aurantium); Utpala (nymphaea stellate); Karpura (cinnamomum camphora); aswatha (ficus religiosa); javitri (myristica fragrance); dronapuspi (leucas cephalotes); murva (marsdenia tenassima); jatiphala (myristica fragrance); citramula (plummbago zeylanica); visamusti (strychnos nuxvomica); kacur (curcuma zedoaria);

Anantamula, sariba (Hemidesmus indicus); apamarga (achyranthes aspera) .;

Amra bija (mangifera indica seeds); Mocarasa (salmalia malabarica);

Cirayata (plumbago zeylanica); bramhadandimula (tricholapsis galaberrinas); suska surana (amrrphophallus compannulatus);

Vamsalochana (bambusa arundinacea); musali (asparagus adscendens);

Bhunimba; karpasa majja (gossypium herbaceum); atibala (abutilon indicum); kurantaka (barleria prionitis); langali (gloriosa superba);

dugdhika (euphorbia prostrta); jalakumbhi (pistia stratiotes);

hribera (coleus vettiveroides); lodhra (symplooas racemosa);

Cangeri (oxalis corniculata); hastidanta (tusk of elephant);

musaparni (teramnus labialis); mundi (sphaeranthus indicus);

Vibhitaki (terminalia belerica); putikaranja (caesalpinia crista);

Arjuna (terminalia arjuna); srivestaka (pinus rosburghi);

Saileya (paramelia perlata); durvamula (datura metel);

Vidari (pueraria tuberose); kapitha (feronia limonia);

Kamala (nelumbo nucifera); padmakha (prunus erasoides);

Karkati- (trapusa cucumis sativus) .; Krishna agaru (aquilaria agallocha);

Vrkshamla (garcinia indica); sankhapushpi (convolvulus pluricaulis);

Brahmi (bacopa maniri); sahadevi (vernonia cinerea);

Girikarnika (clitoria ternatea); mundi (spharnanthus indicus);

Gambhari- (gmelina arborea); kaidarya (bergera koenigh);

Ankola- (alangium salvifolium); cirayita (swertia chirata);

Sakhotaka (streblus aspera); murva (marsdenia tenacissima);

Vishnukranta- (evolvulous alsinoides); mesashringi- (gymnema sylvestre); kucala strychnos nuxvomica; tundi (coccinia indica); suganndhabala; vamsamula (bambusa arundinacea); hastikarni – (arum macrorhizon); padmakha – (prunus cerasoides);

Matyalshi (alternanthera sessilis); girivaluka (wild variety of hrivera); tumburu (zanthoxylumarmatum); gorocana-(bile of oxkankola piper cubeba); ksirakakoli (fritillaria roylei); phalsa (grewiaasiatica); gudamar podapatra-(gymnema sylvestre); madhusnuhi; akuli (cassia obovata); khurasani ajawayin (hyoscymus muticus);

Revandacini (rheum emod); majuphala (quercus infectoria); kanaka puspa (cassia obovata); dhanvayasa (fagonia Arabica); vyaghri (solanumsurattense); saptaparni (alstonia scholaris); cakramarda (cassia tora); sirisa (albizzia lebbeck);

Malati (jasminum arborescens); kancanara; srivestaka (pinus roxburghii); durva (cynodon dactylon); kumara aloe barbadensis; patola (trichosanthes dioica); saliparni desmodiumgangeticum; murva (marsedenia tenacissina); bhumyamalaki (phyllanthus amarus); udumbara (ficus recemosa); saptachad (alstonia scholaris); langali (gloriosa superba); prapoundarika (nelumbo mucifera); syonaka; grandhitagara (valeriona); kakamaci (solanum nigrum); somaraji (psoralia corylofolia); indravaruni (citrullus colocynthis); dusparsa (tragia involucrate); krsnavetra (tiliacora recemosa);

patala (sterospermumsuaveoens); nyagrodha (ficus bengalenses); plaksha (ficus lacor); audumbara (ficus glomerata); karkataka shringi (pistacia chinensis); katu tumbi phala (genaria vulagaris); kulutha (dolichos biflorus); amlavetasa (garcinia pedunculata); nagavalli (piprebetel); meghanada (amaranthus spinusus); lodhra (symplocos racemosa); kadamba (anthocephalus cadamba); plaksha (ficus lacor); vetasa (salix alba); jati (jasminum officinale); harenuka (vitex agnus); katphala (myrica nagi);

vamsatwak (bambusa arundanacea); tumburu (zanthoxylum armatum); granthi tagara (valleriana wallichi); sarapunkha (tephrosia purpurea); ahiphena (papaver somnifeerum); matulungamula (citrus medica); akarakarabha (anacyclus pyrethrum); sarala (pinus roxburghii); dalcini (syzygium); mrddaru shringa (litharge);

Cirayata (swertia chirata); karanja (pongamia pinnata); lodhra (symlocos racemosa); vatankura (ficus bengalenses); kadali musa (paradisiaca); karavellaka (momordica charantia); arka (calotropis procera); bakuci bija (psoralea corylifolia);

katphala (Myrica esculenenta); ketaki (pandanus tectorius); malati (jasminarborescens); talisapatra (abies webbiana); sukti (shell of oyster); kumbhi (careya arborea); kurma prista (external shell of tortoise); kharpara (calamitezincore); devadaru (cedrus deodara); Jayanti (sesbania sesban); Vishnukranta (evolvulus alsinoides); Prisniprni (uraria picta); Atapushpa (aneathum sowa); Kapikacchu (mucuna prurita); Bijapura (cirus medica); Bilwa (aegle marmelos); Agnimantha (clerdendrum phlomedis); Syonaka (roxylumindicum); Gambhari (gmelina arborea); Pathala (stereospermum suaveolens); Kakajangha (Perstrophe bicalyculata); Kundali (azima retracantha);

Sahadevi (vernonia cinerea); Varahikanda (pueraria tuberosa); Plaksha (ficus lacor); Iswari (aristolochia indica); Suddha tankana; karamarda (carissaCaranda; capala (bismuth); suryakshra (potassium nitrate; supari (areca catechu); sringivera sunthi; ankola (alangium salvifolium); sarpakshi (opiorrhiza mungos); pilu (salvadora persica); arka mula (calotropis procera); nilika (indigofera tinctria) .

Karpasa pushpa (gossypium herbaceum); jatiphala (myrista fragrance) jiraka (cuminum cyminum); cavy piper rero fractum; hastikarni (leea macrophylla); malkangini (celastrus paniculatus); sahadevi (vernonia cineria y); yamani (trachyspermum ammi); elavaluka (prunus crerasus); dhatakipuspa (woodfordia fruiticasa); sprikka (anisomeles malabarica); bhang (cannabis sativa); suni sannaka (marsilea minuta); vrscikali (tragiainviucrata); kataka (strychnos potatorum); gawakshimla white clitoria ternatea; hastikarni (colocasia macrorrhiza); nilimula (indigofera tinctoria); granthi tagara; matyakshi (alternanthera sessilis); aparajita (clitoria ternatea); lajjalu (mimosa pudica); samanga –lajjalu; aralu ailanthus excels; cira bilva (holoptelia integrifolia); suranakanda (amorpophallus campanulatus); mundi (sphaeranthus indicus); kankola (piper cubeba); jayanti (leptadenia reticulate) patalgarudi (cocculus hirstus); rajavarta (lapsis lazuli); punnaga (calophyllum inophyllum); hapusha (juniperus communis); ingudi (balanites aegyptiaca); baspikamula (amaranthus bretes); cakramarda (cassia tora); somavalli (ephedra gerardiana); kurantaka (barleria prionitis); riddhi (habenaria intermedia); stauneyak (taxus baccata); sprikka (anisomeles malabarica); satahwa (anethum sowa); tintidika (rhus parviflora); ghotaphala (ziziphus xylopyrus); vrddadaruka (argyreia speciosa); virataru (dichrostchys cineria); musaparni (teramnus labialis); kuberaksha (caesalpinaa bonducella); badramusta (cyperus rotundus); girivalika (wild avoniaodorata); bimbipatra (coccinia indica); urvaruk (cucumis melo); narangi (citrus aurantium); sahadevi (vernonia cinerea); kaseru (scirpus kysoor); babbula (acacia nilotica); agastya (sesbania grandiflora); nagaramotha (cyperus rotundus);

lamajjaka (andropogan); pugiphala (areca catechu); kataka bija (strychnos potatorum);

jatipatri (myristica fragrance); ananasa (ananas comosus); sitalacini (piper cubeba); talamkhana (asteracantha longifolia);

Metals used

Suvarna (Gold); Rajata (silver); Tamra (copper); Loha (iron); Naga (lead); Vanga (tin); Pittala (brass); Kamsya (bronze); Varta (loha any alloy of five metals); parada (mercury); gandhaka (sulphur); Abhraka (biotite mica); Haratala (orpiment); Kasisa (green vitriol; gairika (red ochre); hingula (cinnabara); Manashila (realgar); Sankha (conch); Makshika (chalcopyrite); Tutha (blue vitriol); Giri sindhura (redoxide of mercury); Gauri pashana (white arsenic); Silajitu (mineral pitch;

Sadharana rasa

Kampilla (mallotus philippensis); Samudralavana (seasalt); gauri pshana (white arsenic); Navasadaraammonium chloride); Hingula (cinnabar) agnijara (amber); girisindhura (red oxide of mercury); mriddaru shringa (litharge); Vajra (diamond); Mukta (parl); Pusparaga (topaz); Marakata (emerald); Vaidhurya; Gomeda (hessonite); Manikya (ruby); Nilam (sapphire); Vaikranta (tourmaline);

ANNEXURE 1:

Introduction to Ayurveda

The following is the brief introduction about Ayurveda useful for readers who are quite new to the subject.

आयुरस्मिन् विद्यऽतेनेन वाऽयुर्विन्दतीत्यायुर्वेदः (Su.Su. 1.15) .

हिताहितं सुखं दुःखमायुस्तस्य हिताहितम्|

मानं च तच्च यत्रोक्तमायुर्वेदः स उच्यते||४१|| (ca su 1/41) Ayurveda is science, the subject that deals with life, and by which the long life is achieved is Ayurveda.

It Advocates about Hitayu (advantageous life), Ahita Ayu (disadvantageous life), Sukhayu – happy life, Ahitayu – unhappy life. It also explains what is good and bad for life and yardsticks to measure that for all for these.

समदोषः समाग्निश्च समधातुमलक्रियः |

प्रसन्नात्मेन्द्रियमनाः स्वस्थ इत्यभिधीयते ||४१|| su su 15/41

Ayurvedic definition of health described by Sushruta states in detail that about the factors like the three doshas, agni (metabolic and digestive processes by various enzymes and their interactions, dhatus (tissues), mala (waste products) and their activities are should be in a state of equilibrium, and also normal state of indriya (sense organs), mana (mind) and atma (soul) is considered as health.

Caraka describing the features of lifespan mentions that the decrease of lifespan which is indicated by various sudden abnormal changes occur in the sensory perception, objects of perception, mind, intellect, and movement. These features help in forecasting the remaining lifespan and death of an individual at a particular moment.

Another significant concept is postulating similarities between purusha and loka. It specifies that whatever specific murtimantabhava (embodiments) are present in the loka, the same are in the purusha. Similarly, whatever is in purusha is also in the loka. The collective combination of the six dhatus, viz. prithvi, apa, tejas, vayu, akasha and unmanifested Brahman is labeled as loka (universe) and similar of these six constituents also make the purusha.

Characteristics of the five basic elements i.e Panchmahabhuta which includes space, air, fire, water and earth which form part of both loka and purusha.

Constitution framed by three doshas form the and get associated with human beings right from point of conception in mother's womb. Embryo gets its share of these doshas from sperm of father and ovum of mother. These doshas form constitution (prakriti) of an individual which will be a part of him or her till last breath. This is called dosha prakriti. On other hand, satva, raja and tama form manasa prakriti.

Tri dosha :

Vagbhata describing tridosha and their distribution states that Vayu (Vata), Pitta and Kapha are the three Doshas of the body.

In everyone all three doshas are present but one dosha will be dominant and the other two doshas will be subordinate doshas. Basing on the dosha prakriti and manasa prakriti one exhibita characteristics of the same .

Health depends on the equilibrium of these three doshas and its imbalance leads to diseases.Though Tridosha are present all over the body, but specific sites are stipulated for each of the dosha .

The upper part up to the chest is dominated by Kapha Dosha,

Pitta is dominated by the part between the chest and umbilicus,

The part below the umbilicus is dominated by Vata.

Doshas are made up of panchamahabhuta just as human body too .

Vata is predominant of air and space (vayu and akasa), pitta by fire and water (agni an ap) and kapha by earth and water (prithvi and ap elements respectively) . Integrity and endurance of body depends on integrity of three doshas, hence considered as three pillars of body..

Structural integrity is provided by kapha dosha . This dosha is composed of two elements – prithvi and ap (earth and water) - thus signifying stability. It maintains the body resistance by acting as a cementing agent, giving the body its weight, mass and stability.

Pitta is accountable for heat of body and maintenance of heat is a sign of life. All functions are under the control of pitta. Digestion of food, formation of nutritive juices, segregation of nutrients and wastes, absorption and distribution of nutrients is caused by pitta..

Vata uniformly distributes heat and coldness all through body and balances all physiological activities. Vata controls all functions, it is remote control of every activity of body, and it also controls pitta and kapha, tissues of body and also excretion of wastes. Vata also supervises functions of mind and perception through senses. Vata represents balancing element of body.

Owing to combination of vitiated doshas and weak and susceptible tissues diseases are produced. When doshas undergo vitiation and pass through six stages of pathogenesis, they invade weak and susceptible tissues in fourth stage of pathogenesis (kriyakala) and get lodged therein. This is beginning of disease process. Here, premonitory symptoms of disease would be seen. In the absence of treatment of disease even in this condition, doshas further damage tissues and cause disease with its signs and symptoms in fifth stage of pathogenesis. Progression of the disease to sixth stage of pathogenesis may occur resulting in serious and life threatening complications. In first three stages, doshas undergo accumulation, vitiation and spread to various parts of body. These stages cause dosha disturbances without causing actual disease.

Due to vitiation of rajah tama dosha will be vitiated initially in mental disorders and later vata, pitta and kapha get involved in pathogenesis of disease. Among satva, rajo tamah the quality Satva of mind is not considered as a dosha. In diseases of agantuka nature resulted because of injury (tri doshas get involved in later stages and poduce symptoms of pathogenicity depending on the predominance.

Sattva, Rajas and Tamas are better known as Mansa dosha (Psychic constitution). Precisely, Triguna are known as Ayurvedic mind types.

Similar to tridosha the five elements (Pancha Mahabhutas) are building for Triguna (Sattva, Rajas and Tama) also. In human beings, one or the other Dosha and Guna is dominant either singularly or in combination. Triguna and Tridosha are innately related to each other as they are responsible for an integrated personality composition at the physical and psychological level.

Sattva Guna is marked by positive attitude, happiness, lightness, spiritual connection and consciousness. Sattvic state is defined as disease free body. Sattva arouses the senses and represents intellect and knowledge.

Rajas Guna is supposed to be active among trigunas and characterised by stimulation and motion. Passion and eager for achievement are outcome of Rajas Guna.

Tamas Guna has two powerful characters i.e. resistance and heaviness. It stimulates negative thoughts in the mind and induces lethargy, sleep and apathy.

Agni:

Agni is another important concept of Ayurveda, and the term Agni is used in the sense of digestion of food and metabolic products. So it is the great source of energy in universe as well as in the body. Consumed food is to be digested, absorbed and assimilated, which is essential for the maintenance of life performed by Agni. As Charaka mentions that the individual dies once the cessation of the function of Agni occurs, and equilibrium state of agni keeps the individual healthy and would lead a long, happy and enjoys disease free life. But, in its deranged state the whole metabolism would be disturbed, resulting in ill health. Hence, Agni is said to be the base (mool) of life. Jatharagni is vital one among thirteen types of Agni, viz, - Jatharagni, seven Dhatwagnis and five Bhutagnis, controlling all other agnis through its power.

Sapta dhatu:

The human body is primarily made up of Saptadhatus and is responsible for the entire structure of the body. The dhatus maintain the functioning of different systems, organs and vital parts of the body and play a major role in the development and nourishing of the body.

With the help of agni (fire), Dhatus are responsible for the immune processes thus play a vital role in the protective mechanism of the body. Each tissue or dhatu is primarily governed by one of the tridoshas – vata, pitta & kapha. When one dhatu is defective, its impact will be on successive dhatu, as each dhatu receives its nourishment from the dhatu proceeding to it. The seven dhatus are described here as follows.

Rasa, rakta, mamsa, medas, asthi, majjja and shukra are called dhatus beacause, they support the body.

As per Susruta the transformation of Rasa dhatu rakta gets formed, then from raktamamsa gets formed, from mamsa medas is formed, from medas asthi is formed and from asthi majja is formed from majja shukra gets formed.

1) Rasa (Plasma) is the first dhatu and contains nutrients & minerals from digested food and nourishes & replenishes all the tissues and organs.

2) Rakta (blood) transports oxygen to all tissues and vital organs and thus maintains life.

3) Mamsa (muscle) which covers vital organs, and enables movements of bones & joints and maintains the physical capacity and strength of the body.

4) Meda (Adipose tissue) maintains the lubrication and oiliness of all the tissues.

5) Asthi (bones and Cartilage) gives support to the body structure.

6) Majja (bone marrow) fills up the bony spaces

7) Shukra, which are the reproductive tissues responsible for reproduction. Sperm in males and Ova in females.

The vitiated doshas directly affect dhatus, thus vitiated dhatus initiate the disease process. Once we identify the root cause of the illness is known, therapies administered accordingly to balance the system through reducing the excess element (s) and increasing the deficient one (s) . Maintaining the balance of the dhatus by keeping tridoshas in equilibrium through a proper diet, exercise and recovery program.

Concept of Vyadhikshamatwam described in Charaka Samhitha relates to Immunity. Immunity is the ability of the body to overcome and resist diseases. According to Ayurveda, Ojas is considered to be the dhatu Sara essence of tissue essential to keep up Optimum Health. If the Ojas is destroyed, the human being will also perish.

Concept of Ojas: Ojas is the purest, finest essence formed from all seven dhatu. And that itself is bala according to Ayurveda.

Oja is circulated all over the body with Rasa dhatu and rakta dhatu through ojovaha sira. These channels originate from the heart (mahata).

Ojas is nourished from the nutrient fluid (ahara rasa) as like other dhatu.

Functions:

Two types of functions are mentioned for both ojases

1) **Para ojas:** Ojas forms the beginning of the formation of the embryo. It is the essential nourishing fluid developed from the rasas of the embryo. It enters the heart right at the stage of the latter's initial formation and is permanently located there; sustain the life of the foetus.

Loss of ojas amounts to to the loss of life itself.

Oja is present in two forms: supreme (para) and mediocre (apara). The supreme form (para ojas) is the most important component responsible for the vitality of life. Its quantity in the body is measured as eight drops (bindu). It is located in the heart. It is generally stable in the body in an equilibrium state. Destruction of this component can cause death.

Ahara parinama

Ahara maintains and supports deha dhatus, Ojas, Bala and Varna with the help of Agni. Hence in Ayurveda, Ahara is considered as one among the Trayopastambha. The ingested Ahara has to get digested to undergo absorption. Every food particles should undergo different stages of digestion in order to convert macronutrients into micro particles to aid easy absorption. Factors like Agni, Ahara Parinamakara Bhavas, Ahara Vidhi Visheshayatana and Ahara Sevana Vidhi contributes to this process. Hence, all these factors collectively maintain the process of digestion leading to Utpatti of Prakruta Dosha thereby achieving Dhatu Poshana.

There are prime four Dhatu Poshan Nyaya's described by Acharya's. They are as follows.

1. Ksheeradadhi Nyaya – (Theory of complete Transformation process) According to this theory the Poorva dhatu is completely converted into Uttara dhatu as like the milk is totally converted in to curd, the curd into butter and the butter into ghee.

2. Kedarkulya Nyaya – (Theory of Transportation process)

According to this Nyaya, the meaning of kedari is paddy or wheat field and kulya means canal. Just like the distribution of water from river, well or tank to plot in rice or wheat field through a main channel to supply water to the nearest as to the farthest plots one after one

3. Khalekapot Nyaya – (Theory of Selection process)

The term "Khala" means the field where the grains are fallen after cutting the crop and Kapota means the pigeons. Thus According to Khale Kapot Nyaya, the pigeons coming from different place and distance to pick up the kind of grains they need and return to their own place residing either early or late depending upon the distance and direction they require to travel

4. Ek kaal dhatuposhan Nyaya – (Dynamic process)

According to this Nyaya, Ahara rasa nourishes all dhatus at the same time by their Dhatuvaha strotas.

Atma and ayu

Ayu (Life) is state of union of as Atma (conciousness), Sharir (physical body), Indriya (sensory and motor organs) Satva (Mana) . When all these factors are in conjugation then only there is life. Life is the extension of consciousness; means the life span is the time period upto which there is presence of Atma.

Shad dhatu Purush is the combination of Panchmahabhoot and Chetna. Atma is responsible for consciousness hence also called as Chetana dhaatu .

Thus indriya acts as mediators in revealing the symptoms of life by Atma. They stand as differentiating factors between the sendriya or chetana (sentient) and nirindriya or achetana (non-sentient) matters.

सेन्द्रियं चेतनं द्रव्यं, निरिन्द्रियमचेतनम्॥ (ca su 1/48) .

Indriyas are the basic component or instruments in differentiating the living and non-living matters.

Purushasya vishaya jnanartham.... Visesho va indriya- su sa 1

Indriyas are the specific factors or organs situated in body and act as means for acquiring the knowledge of various objects and performing various activities of the body.

Mana: The one object responsible for thinking, contemplating or knowledge is called as satva or Mana.

It is responsible for having all pleasure full feelings sukha.

It is also called as atindriya as it helps to know everything when it connects the indriyas to their respective sense or matter.

It is also called as satva.

Srotas:

The internal transport system of the body, represented by srotasas, has been given a place of fundamental importance in Ayurveda-both in health and disease. No structure in the body can grow and develop or waste and atrophy, independent of stoases that transport seven dhatus, which latter are constantly subjected to transformation. There mainly thirteen in number.apart from this dojo, mano, sajnavaha, chestavaha sorts are described. Sort dusty causes disease.

Tri Malas:

In Ayurveda much information is given with respect to Malas .The three major excreta of the body are the waste products of metabolism. These are Pureesha (stools), Mutra (urine), Sweda (sweat) .

These three are formed continually and keep the body fit and healthy and get excreted out of the body at proper time and in right quantity. Otherwise they get retained in the body and produce many diseases.

Ashtanga Ayurveda (The Eight Limbs of Ayurveda) :

The description of Ashtanga Ayurveda shows the existence of the 'knowledge of branches of a science' in the olden days. It also gives us a clue that the art of studying and graduating in different branches of the same science under different teachers.

कायबालग्रहोध्वाङ्ग शल्यदंष्ट्रा जरावृषान् || अष्टावङ्गानि तस्याहुः चिकित्सा येषु संश्रिता | (As su 1/5, 6)

Ashtanga Ayurveda refers to the eight limbs of Ayurveda. Ayurveda, originally known as great Indian seers into divided Ashtanga Ayurveda destine eight branches.

Kayachikitsa (internal medicine

Shalya tantra- surgery

Shalakya Tantra (disease above the clavicle) Shalakya deals with the diseases of the eyes, ear, nose and throat.

Kaumara Bhritya (paediatrics)

Agad Tantra; Agad Tantra deals with natural and artificial toxic substances and poisons in detail along with their antidotes, the signs and symptoms and also the management of poisoning resulting from the bites of animals like snakes, insects, spiders, rodents. Vyavharayurveda (jurisprudence) is integral part of Agad Tantra.

Rasayana. Rasayana is a substance used for promoting rasa and allied tissues (saptdhatu of Ayurveda) .

Vajikarana The drugs etc. which induce euphoria in sexual activity of male partner thereby performs like a horse is known as vajikarana

Diagnosis:

A comprehensive clinical examination is the basis for proper diagnosis of a disease. A proper diagnosis of the disease is the basis for planning a proper treatment protocol.

According to Ayurveda, the clinical examination is twofold. It should be methodically done including these two stages of examination. They are as below mentioned.

Basic clinical examination in Ayurveda carried oiut mainly in 2 ways.

Roga Pareeksha & roga pariksha

1. Roga Pariksha (disease examination)

The disease should be examined to know –

The quality and nature of the disease (adibala, janmabala, doshabala pravritta etc.) aggressive and complicatory state of the disease. It is mainly studied under five headings. Nidana (causes of the disease); Poorvarupa (symptoms which occur before the manifestation of the disease); (rupa) Signs and symptoms of the disease .

Upashaya-Anupashaya (Aggravating and pacifying factors of the disease); Samprapti (the process of formation of the disease); Saadhya-Asaadhyata (curability and incurability of the disease); upadrava (Complications and Sequel of a disease) .

Rogi Pareeksha (patient examination) :

Rogi Pareeksha should be done to know

Prakriti (Basic constitution); Vikriti – (pathological changes occur in the body);

Sara (quality and quantity of the tissues); Samhanana (Compactness of the body); Pramana – Measurements of the body parts (normal and abnormal caliculations of the body

Satmya – (Compatibilities to body which are conducive to the health).

Satwa – Mental strength, (emotions and moods of the patient)

Ahara Shakti – (Assessment of metabolism)

Vyayama Shakti – (Exercise tolerance)

Vaya (Age of patient which gieves informations about dose and probable disorders)

Bala -Physical built strength and immunity of the patient.

There are many ways in which Rogi Pareeksha or examination of the patient is conducted. Among them trividha pariksha (pratyaksham (as seen and perceived by doctor directly), sanumanam (Inference), aptopadesa (advise by the elders and sastra), shadvidha parikasha (6 fold diagnosis)

Chakshurindriya pareeksha – examination by seeing (inspection)

Ghranendriya pareeksha – examination through smelling

Shravanendriya pareeksha – examination through hearing (auscultation)

Jihvendriya pareeksha – examination through taste

Sparshanendriya pareeksha – examination through touch

Prashna pareeksha – interrogation. Another important examination is Ashta Sthana Pareeksha.Ashta Sthana Pareeksha (8 fold diagnosis) includes examination of nadi (pulse), mala (stool), mootra (urine), jihwa (tongue), shabda (sounds), sparsha (touch), drik (eye), akriti (built, gait, decubits etc).

Dashavidha Pareeksha is also been advised to assess the strength of the patient to decide dose and also to assess the curability and incurability of the disease in him.

Treatment:

The balance state and proper functioning of Doshas, Dhatus, Srotas and Agni, etc. provide good health status and achievement of this is the prime concern of Ayurveda therapies.

The therapeutic principle in Ayurveda based on several things which includes pacification of Doshas, potentiation of Dhatus, restoring functioning of Agni, cleaning the obstruction of Srotas and preventing formation of Ama, etc. Ayurveda therapies, can be broadly categorizes into three major classes.

1.Daivavyapashraya Chikitsa:

It is non-pharmacological therapy based on faith in God or worship and rituals. This therapy commonly practices in case of emergency or poisoning condition and also practiced in ancient time when other approaches where yet to evolved. Chanting of Mantra and Japa are major practices comes under Daivavyapashraya Chikitsa. The faith in Daiva or divine power is the only basis of this therapy. This therapy utilizes practices of Daana means being charitable, conduction of Homa as cleansing measures with the help of fire element and Suraarchanais means uses of power of prayer. This therapy directly or indirectly influences Manas, reduces stress and enhances inner strength.

2. Sattvavajaya Chikitsa:

This therapy mainly utilizes for mental illness and used as psycho-behavioral therapy. This therapy helps to controls Krodha, Kama, Bhay, Moha, Lobha, Irsha, Visada and Dwesa. These all elements are considered as causes of mental illness and Sattvavajaya Chikitsa helps to control these factors thus provides relief in stress, anxiety anddepression, etc. Sattvavajaya makes mind positive and aggressive emotions. Various approaches in this therapy can be employed to inculcate positive Gyana, Vigyana, Dhairya, Smriti and Samadhi.

3. Yuktivyapashraya Chikitsa:

Yuktivyapashraya is logical or rationale approach of disease management based on the types of diseases and requirements of patient's conditions. This therapy mainly encompasses two types of treatments internal as well as external therapies. Langhan, Brumhan, Shodhan and Shaman therapies, etc.are major treatment regimen of Yuktivyapashraya.

Shodhan, Samsham and Langhan treatments reduce aggravated Kapha Dosha and Brumhan therapy controls vitiated Vata and Pitta dosha. Shodhan therapy removes vitiated Doshas from the body, which includes therapeutic procedures like Vaman and Virechana etc., panchakarma.

Samshaman therapy alleviates vitiated Doshas with the help of medicines and dietary control. Atapsevan, Vyayama, Trusha, Vayusevan, Deepan, Pachan and helps to controls these factors thus provides relief in stress, anxiety and

Kshudhadharana etc. Are examples of Samshaman therapy. The drugs of various properties used for specific disease depending upon the stage of pathological manifestations. The Rasa and Guna of herbal medicines offers particular therapeutic advantages thus drugs selected on the basis of their properties i.e. Rasa, Guna, Virya and Vipaka etc.

General Classification of Chikitsa: Nidanparivarjan It states avoidance of causative factors which may leads disequilibrium of Doshas, Dhatu & Mala thus initiates Samprapti of the disease

Rasayana and vajikarana chikitsa:

This therapy utilizes Rasayan and Vajikaran drugs, amongst them Rasayan drugs used for the rejuvenation purpose and Vajikaran drugs used to enhances sexual vigor. Rasayan & Vajikaran therapies serve as preventive measure and also used for treating some diseases.

Rogprashaman treatments applied to cure the disease but in this case chances of recurrence of disease still persisted.

Apunarbhava chikitsa: It prevents recurrence of the disease and provides relief from cardinal symptoms

Dravyabhoota chikitsa: It includes all therapeutics measures which used to treat different types diseases.

Adravyabhoot chikitsa: It resembles methods used to cure diseases other than common therapeutics approaches; this may includes Vismapan, Vyayam and Upavas.

Daivavyapashray refers to the faith healing or methods have a religious reasoning for curing diseases. Mantra, Jap and Homa etc. are common ways of spiritual healing. Yuktivyapashray refers to the approaches for treating disease as per the condition of patient and progressive stage of disease. Combinations of medicines, consideration of age of patient, severity of the disease and dietary regimen all comes under this heading.

Satvawaya resembles psycological treatment; this treatment not only provides mental benefits but also helps to cure physical illness.

Ayurveda described some conducts which are to be followed for maintaininghealthy well being. Pathyapathya, Brahmacharya, Dincharya, Ritucharya and Sadvritta, etc. are suggestive conducts of Ayurveda, which helps in the maintenance of general health.

Ayurveda described Ahara, Nidra and Brahmacharya as sub-pillars of life, the suggestive dietary and daily regimen helps lot to combat against any disease. Waking up early, eating healthy foods, fruits and vegetables, avoidance of late night awakening andconsiderations of concept ofPathya and Apathya gives immense health benefits and prevents diseases.

Dincharya (daily regimen) and Ritucharya (seasonal regimen) also boost natural immunity thus provides resistance against common infections and improves inner strength. Sadvritta and Achara Rasayana imparts values of good moral and social conducts thus boost mental strength and combat against pathogenesis of mental disorders.

The therapeutic procedures of Ayurveda control vitiated Doshas, reverse depletion of Dhatus, potentiate functioning of Agni and detoxify body by facilitating excretion of Mala thus helps to treat many physical and mental diseases.

APPENDIX

Abhicara jwara, 67

abhraka, 9, 15, 101, 103, 114, 157, 168, 169, 171, 172

Abhraka, 168, 169, 171, 262

ABHRAKA, 167

About the book, 4

Agantuka asta jwara, 80

ahika jwara, 90

Ahika jwara, 90

amajwara, 74

anupana, 8, 15, 66, 75, 76, 124, 143, 149, 151, 154, 157, 165, 167, 173, 177, 179, 187, 189, 215, 236, 247

Anupana, 151, 236

astajwara santi, 105

bhudhara yantra, 16, 199

Bhudhara yantra, 199

dhatugata jwara, 55

Dhatugata jwara, 77

dola yantra, 16, 172, 181, 186, 188, 229

Dola yantra, 181, 200, 201

dosage of bhasma, 176

Dosage of Bhasma, 176

doshahetuka jwara, 56

examination of tongue, 49

examination of urine, 48

gandhaka, 13, 14, 15, 19, 89, 90, 91, 93, 99, 101, 116, 123, 124, 125, 141, 148, 158, 159, 163, 164, 166, 167, 169, 174, 177, 179, 197, 198, 201, 217, 218, 219, 220, 221, 224, 226, 230, 234, 235, 262

Gandhaka, 114, 123, 166, 167, 198, 218

Gandharva jwara, 69

garbha yantra, 16, 196

hingulam, 90, 91, 92, 93, 101, 102, 103, 104

Hingulam, 174

jala yantra, 16, 197

Jwara dinacharya, 61, 62

jyotissastrabhipraya, 115

kacchapa yantra, 197

Kacchapa yantra, 196

kanta bhasma, 158, 230

karmavipaka, 6, 11, 1, 7, 13, 14, 15, 17, 18, 19, 20, 26, 31, 106, 119, 138

Karmavipaka, 8, 9, 10, 11, 12, 14, 15, 16, 17, 18, 19, 20, 21,

23, 25, 26, 27, 28, 29, 30, 31, 32, 119

Kasa jwara, 76

Krimi jwara, 70

Lohabhasma pariksha, 158

Magadha prastha, 16, 206

manahshila, 177

Manahshila, 175

murcha jwara, 79

Murcha jwara, 79

panchakarma, 6, 238, 240, 241, 242, 243, 244, 278

Panchakarma, 238, 239, 240, 241

patala yantra, 16

Patala yantra, 201

pathya and apathya, 15, 241

Pathya and apathya, 90, 245

PATHYA AND APATHYA, 23

Pisaca jwara, 68

puta, 16, 148, 149, 153, 166, 188, 189, 191, 192, 193, 198, 203, 204, 205, 224, 234

Puta, 149, 174, 203

rakta mokshana, 207, 242, 243

rasakarpoora, 132, 165, 187

Rasakarpoora, 165, 187

roupya, 151, 179, 198

Roupya, 150, 151, 171

sannipata jwara, 20, 85, 97, 98

Sannipata jwara, 93, 98

silajitu, 15, 157, 181, 182

Silajitu, 142, 157, 181, 182, 262

tamra, 13, 15, 90, 91, 99, 101, 104, 116, 124, 125, 147, 152, 176, 177, 218, 222, 234, 237

Tamra, 13, 152, 176, 177, 217, 262

tanka yantra, 16

tridosa, 44

upadhatu, 15, 178

Upadhatu, 178

vajra, 16, 74, 153, 187, 188, 189, 190, 192, 193, 199, 231

Vajra, 168, 188, 189, 190, 192, 262

vajra musa, 192, 199

valuka yantra, 16, 163, 201

Valuka yantra, 195

Vamana jwara, 74

vanga, 15, 99, 103, 147, 150, 151, 153, 161, 178

Vanga, 153, 154, 181, 262

vatavyadhi, 8, 128

Vatavyadhi, 8, 9, 125, 131, 190

vidhyadhara yantra, 16

Vidhyadhara yantra, 194

vimsati kshaya, 108

visama jwara, 79

Visama jwara, 79

www.ingramcontent.com/pod-product-compliance
Lightning Source LLC
LaVergne TN
LVHW061608070526
838199LV00078B/7206